D1272173

Back pain

THE FACTS

MALCOLM I. V. JAYSON
Rheumatic Diseases Centre
University of Manchester

Line drawings
by
Richard Neave

OXFORD
OXFORD UNIVERSITY PRESS
NEW YORK TORONTO
1981

Oxford University Press, Walton Street, Oxford OX2 6DP
London Glasgow New York Toronto
Delhi Bombay Calcutta Madras Karachi
Kuala Lumpur Singapore Hong Kong Tokyo
Nairobi Dar es Salaam Cape Town
Melbourne Wellington
and associate companies in
Beirut Berlin Ibadan Mexico City

British Library Cataloguing in Publication Data

Jayson, Malcolm I.V.
Back pain. — (Oxford medical publications)
1. Backache
I. Title
616.7'3   RD768
ISBN 0-19-261285-9

Set by Hope Services, Abingdon
Printed in Great Britain by
Richard Clay (The Chaucer Press) Ltd,
Bungay, Suffolk

Foreword

by

CHARLES PHELPS

Chelsea College, University of London

Last summer, I 'slipped a disc'. I could not point to any immediate incident as a cause; I woke one morning with some
discomfort in one leg and when I got up I found that I could
not move freely. I felt particularly aggrieved because this was
at a time when I was hoping to tidy my mother's house prior
to sale and to build a wall in the garden of my own house. I
soon found these had to be abandoned. After a little wifely
nagging, I went to the doctor who examined me and gave the
curiously euphemistic diagnosis: I had a 'slipped' disc.

I tell this not because I wish to excite sympathy, but to
produce my credentials for joining the club of 'back pain
sufferers'. Quite apart from the restrictive physical practices
to which I had to become accustomed, there were other per-
plexities. Why the smile when I hobbled into a room? There
was a faint but unmistakable suggestion that I was a species
of malingerer and that my problems could not possibly be as
incommoding as I made out.

It was the first time I had been stricken with anything that
changed the quality of my life. Now there were things I
could and could not do physically. The advice I was given
made it clear this was not something that would get better in
the timescale of recovery from 'flu: about a year, if I took
care of myself, I was told.

The other feature I noted was that unless I wanted to
shackle myself in hospital, self-help was the order of the day.
Where did this start? For me, in trying to understand what
had gone wrong. Perhaps man travelled through the evolutionary time scale too rapidly from his happily buoyant position
in water through the stability of a four-legged design on dry
land to this two-legged defiance of gravity, and therefore we

v

Foreword

all have a cryptic tendency to structural failure. Whatever the story, I would recommend this excellent book by Professor Jayson for all who wonder at the disabling nature of these human structural disorders. A knowledge of the cause of the problem predisposes the sufferer to adopt postures (both physical and mental) that can intelligently aid the process of recovery.

It is fashionable to believe that most diseases have an explanation ultimately revealing a fault at the molecular level. There is ample evidence for such a belief when we come to study, for instance, some hereditary diseases and a number of bacterial ailments. It is altogether more difficult to travel along a reductionist pathway in explaining the failure of structural systems, and the reason for this is implicit in the word *systems*. Just as it would be difficult to produce, *intact*, the individual elements from a prestressed concrete girder, so it is not yet possible (and may never be) to reconstruct the working physiological system from the assortment of specific molecules of which it is composed.

Research has produced an abundant understanding of what goes to make up the connective tissues of the body. The molecular components have been minutely described and the geography of their occurrence in tissues such as intervertebral discs of cartilage is well understood. A start has been made in modelling connective tissue, in an attempt to understand how the particular blend of components can in one mixture make bone, whilst in another cartilage or intervertebral disc. The analogy with the prestressed girder can be pursued: the dry cement and sand and steel reinforcements correspond to the molecular components of a tissue. When water is mixed and certain spatial arrangements are made, a girder can become capable of supporting structures, which neither concrete nor steel alone would do. It is when we come to do this reconstruction process with our biological systems that we cannot yet claim success, and one of the most exciting areas of research is finding out why we cannot reproduce the properties of the whole from the sum of the parts.

Foreword

I spend a good part of my scientific life attempting to solve problems such as I have just posed. I and the countless number of other research workers here and abroad recognize the importance of fundamental enquiry and thereby the need for money in supporting the experiments which must be set up. In the case of back pain charitable trusts in the United Kingdom deserve special mention and bodies such as the Arthritis and Rheumatism Council, the Nuffield and Wellcome Trusts all have generously supported what may often have looked like inauspicious ventures. Just as the molecules that make up the system are diverse, so are the talents of the research investigators. It is a marvellous human meeting-ground of, among others: engineers, surgeons, physicians, immunologists, anatomists, biophysicists, and biochemists, from whose committed perseverance to the problems of skeletal disorders come spin-offs additional to those of pure science. Because of such multidisciplinary research, the secretary sits a little more comfortably in her chair, the orthopaedic aids are a little better designed, and new materials for hip replacements appear.

But progress in research is gradual, as is recovery from these disabilities, so we should not expect overnight miracles. However, the optimism that all good scientists have must surely see to it that the presently intractable problems of back pain are eventually solved.

Preface

Back pain is so common and widespread that it is no exaggeration to say that nearly everybody suffers from it sooner or later. It is very difficult to comprehend the immensity of the problem, as back pain occurs at all ages and in all levels of society. More days off work are lost because of back troubles than for almost any other reason and this is so not only for the manual labourer but also for those with relatively 'soft' jobs, such as office executives.

Pain in the back is not a new phenomenon. Studies of skeletons from archeological remains show precisely the same types of change that occur today. The writings of the ancient Greek physicians describe very similar problems and indeed some of their forms of treatment are not so very different from those that we still use. Even examination of the skeletons of animals such as the enormous dinosaur in the Natural History Museum in London reveals similar types of wear and tear in the spine.

Although the back problem has been known for such a long time it is only quite recently that its importance has emerged and we have begun to appreciate the amount of suffering and the economic burden it produces. Increasingly the medical profession is asked how to prevent the development of back pain, how to pick out those who are likely to suffer from it, and the best forms of treatment. As soon as we start to ask these questions we realize that not all back pains are the same and that this sympton can develop for many different reasons. Some of these are clear cut and obvious but in many instances we are unable to sort out the precise cause of the trouble in the individual sufferer.

Modern science is increasingly aware of the need for further research in this field and the subject is of interest not only to physicians and surgeons but also pathologists, radiologists, psychologists, biochemists, bioengineers, and many other disciplines. In the long run, the only way to achieve real advances is a proper understanding of what causes the pain and why it has happened. Often opinions are expressed, particularly by non-medical practitioners, that are not based upon scientific fact but rather on personal concepts which have not been tested in an acceptable way. Many of the myths that surround the whole subject arise because such views are put forward didactically and without the critical self-examination that is normally expected in medical circles. This lax approach applies equally to the many forms of treatment used for back sufferers. No acknowledgement is made of the fact that most episodes of back pain improve or get completely better spontaneously. It is a bit like having a cold and taking a medicine X: even though X is completely valueless, one can be sure that the cold will get better within a week or so. Many claims are made for the efficacy of various types of treatment without appreciating the natural improvements and fluctuations in the pain that normally occur. Individual anecdotal stories of dramatic improvements after different types of treatment abound, yet studies to demonstrate their true effectiveness can tell a very different story. The persistence of the back problem, despite all the claims made, points to the considerable difficulties with which we are faced. I firmly believe in the identification of the cause of the back pain in the individual and prescribing and determining the values of the appropriate forms of treatment for that particular problem. Modern ideas about pain and its control help us to understand and develop various types of treatment to control pain irrespective of the cause. Although this approach is very helpful in relieving symptoms it cannot solve the problem, as the basic causes are not tackled.

Advice for the back sufferer is plentiful. This book has been written to give the reader deeper insight into the whole problem. It endeavours to explain current views on the causes of back pain and the significance of the various changes that occur in the spine. I have described the various types of treatment that are in common use and reviewed whether they

really work. It does seem possible to minimize the back problem with postural and ergonomic advice and this also is
included.

Back pain is the commonest form of rheumatism and its
control is the biggest challenge in rheumatology. A proper
understanding of what is happening is crucial for further
medical advances. I hope that this book will be of help to
back sufferers and stimulate further interest in the topic.

Rheumatic Diseases Centre   *Malcolm I. V. Jayson*
University of Manchester   *February 1981*

Contents

To Judi, Gordon, and Robs

1

Structure and function of the human spine

During evolution the animal kingdom split into two main groups: the invertebrates and the vertebrates. The invertebrates possess no internal skeleton but instead have a tough outer shell or exo-skeleton. The various parts of the limbs and trunk articulate with one another and movement is provided by muscles attached on the inside of this outer case. Such a structure is found in countless species, including insects and shellfish. In some the exo-skeleton has become thick and tough, providing protection for the internal tissues and acting as a suit of armour. However, the rigidity of this system produces considerable problems. For example a rigid system such as this cannot accommodate growth. A change of skeleton must take place at regular intervals. The very nature of the joints between rigid segments allows the animal to produce stereotyped movements but severely restricts its ability to adapt and evolve in relation to altered environmental conditions. These constraints have left the invertebrates relatively lowly members of the animal kingdom.

In contrast the vertbrates have an internal skeleton. In the trunk there is a backbone or vertebral column and in the limbs the various long bones. This skeleton grows with the animal and is flexible, as its components are connected by various types of joints designed according to the requirements at each site. Muscles, ligaments, and other structures are attached to this internal skeleton and can produce a subtlety and complexity of movements that are lacking in invertebrates. This type of structure can be seen in primitive animals such as the lancet, coelacanth, and even the modern dogfish. Natural selection has allowed the more successful species to flourish at the expense of those less well adapted to their environment. This process of evolution has led to the development of modern species of fish, amphibians, reptiles, birds, and mammals. The internal skeletons of all these diverse groups show similar fundamental structures but with extreme adaptations to the species' way of life.

Nearly all animals walk on all four limbs with the trunk horizontal. Man is almost unique in standing upright balanced on two limbs. The advantages of this posture are obvious but clearly it also leads to considerable stresses on the skeleton. This alone could be responsible for many of the back problems that we suffer today. That is not to say that animals do not suffer from backache. Communication is difficult but we do know that dachshunds with their long and relatively poorly supported spines are very prone to this problem.

It has been argued that if the upright posture were responsible for producing spinal problems, natural selection would not have favoured the vertical position and we would all be walking on four legs. However, the span of life during effectively all the period of man's evolution was only some 20 to 30 years. As the majority of back problems occur at an older age, back pain would hardly affect the evolutionary process.

The functions of the human spine

The backbone or vertebral column is the principal supporting structure in the human body. Both upper and lower limbs are attached to it through a complex series of joints. The ribs are attached to the spine in the back of the chest wall in such a way that contraction of muscles allows co-ordinated expansion of the chest and breathing. Muscles, ligaments, and tendons connect various parts of the spine to each other and other structures, allowing a wide variety of movements.

In order to see the structure of the vertebral column, one can do no better than look at the work of Andreas Vesalius. He was an anatomist born in Brussels and was professor in Louvain and Pavia. He produced a magnificent book in 1543 entitled *De Humani Corporis Fabrica* – The Structure of the Human Body. This was a new departure in the study of

2

Structure and function of the human spine

FIG. 1. The human skeleton. Illustration from *De Humani Corporis Fabrica* by Andreas Vesalius (1543)

anatomy, as it was based entirely on dissection. This volume is remarkable for its illustrations by Italian draughtsmen. There is a large series of plates that illustrate human anatomy in superb detail. One of the joys of these drawings is the sense of emotion in the postures of the subjects. Many of the plates include a background against which the subject is posed and the separate plates can be joined together to give a panoramic view of Tuscany in the sixteenth century.

The spine has to carry a heavy load. At any level it is the vertebral column which is principally responsible for transmitting the weight of the body above and any loads being lifted or carried. When muscles contract to produce movements or stabilize joints, there is often additional stress on the vertebral column. The spine is, however, remarkably flexible. It can bend forwards, backwards, and sideways and it can twist. Often these movements are undertaken in complex combinations and with load-bearing at the same time.

The spinal cord emerges from the base of the brain and passes downwards through the vertebral column. It subdivides into nerve roots which emerge through spaces between the vertebrae. These nerves will reach virtually every body tissue. They carry information from the tissues to the spinal cord and then to the brain, allowing perception of sensations. In turn messages from the brain are carried back down the spinal cord and along the nerves to activate muscles and produce movements. The spinal cord is an extremely delicate and complicated structure. It is protected against damage by lying within a column of bony arches in the back of the spine. This is known as the vertebral canal. The nerve roots separate from the spinal cord and pass obliquely downwards to emerge from the vertebral canal through openings known as intervertebral foramina. Despite the complex movements undertaken by the spine, normally no damage to the spinal cord or nerve roots will arise.

Apart from the structural functions of the vertebral column is the requirement that it should function for a lifetime of perhaps 70 or 80 years or even more. With all the wonders of

FIG. 2. The vertebral column, spinal cord, and nerve roots

5

modern science are there any man-made materials that could stand up to such use for that period of time? Can modern designers and engineers produce comparable structures that would still work after all those years? Our cars have problems after two or three years and their average life is only about twelve to fourteen years.

In children the spine is flexible and supple whereas in the elderly it usually has become stiff and much more unyielding. What are the changes that take place and why do they occur? Do they inevitably accompany growing older? Are these changes the cause of back pain and is back pain inevitable? Are there ways of preventing these changes or are current forms of treatment merely tinkering with the problems?

In this book the things that can go wrong in the back and the ways they may produce pain will be described. There is much to be learned and it must be admitted that the study of back pain is still in its infancy. A lot has been written about the changes that occur but often these are personal opinions and have not or cannot be substantiated. It is only relatively recently that detailed studies of the structure and function of the human spine, of what can go wrong, how back pain is produced, and testing of the true values of different forms of treatment have been undertaken. Progress is slow but real for all that. It is the purpose of this book to give a factual account of the current position and the ways forward in the future.

The vertebral column

We all think of man as being upright and indeed sometimes apply moral values to this posture! However, simple observation will show that the spine is not straight but has a number of curves. The low back or lumbar region is slightly hollowed so that it is curved backwards. This is known technically as the lumbar lordosis. The back of the chest is curved slightly forwards and the neck points slightly forwards. In the various problems that arise in the spine this normal pattern may change. The curves may be lost or exaggerated. There may be

Structure and function of the human spine

cervical
vertebrae

dorsal or
thoracic
vertebrae

lumbar
vertebrae

pelvis

sacrum

FIG. 3. The vertebrae of the spine

an abnormal curvature forwards — a kyphosis, a sideways twist — a scoliosis, or there may be a sharp kink. Not only do these abnormal postures develop due to various types of disease, but also they may make things worse by altering the ways in which the spine works and placing stresses on parts of the spine not designed to deal with them.

The spine consists of a column of bony blocks known as vertebrae standing one on top of the other. In the neck there are seven which are known as cervical vertebrae; there are twelve in the back of the chest — the dorsal or thoracic vertebrae; and five in the back — the lumbar vertebrae. The bottom or fifth lumbar vertebra (L5) is directly attached to the sacrum or tail bone. The sacrum is the back part of the pelvis, a ring of bone providing support for the spine and trunk.

All the vertebrae have similar basic structures but with considerable variations at each level, reflecting the different functions at each site. For example the neck is remarkably flexible and only has to bear the weight of the skull. The cervical vertebrae are very lightly built and shaped so as to allow a considerable range of movement between them. In contrast the back has to bear the weight of the trunk and transmits forceful movements of the body. The lumbar vertebrae are much thicker and tougher structures with relatively limited movements allowed between them.

Each vertebra consists of a cylindrical part in front known as the vertebral body. This has flat upper and lower surfaces known as the vertebral end-plates. The vertebral body is convex in the front and flattened behind. This flattened area forms the front part of the canal down which the spinal cord and nerve roots pass. The vertebral arch surrounds the rest of the canal giving protection to the structures within. Each vertebra is joined to those above and below by joints between the vertebral bodies and between the arches.

The intervertebral disc lies between the vertebral end-plates. It is a cushion of tissue that normally provides a springy and movable connection between the bones. Three types of movement occur at this cushion — flattening under loads, bending,

8

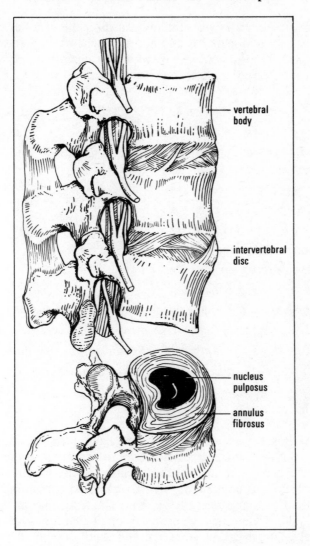

FIG. 4. The vertebrae and intervertebral disc

and twisting. However, unlike a cushion the disc has a very definite structure that is all-important when things go wrong. Basically the disc consists of two parts: a central area known as the nucleus pulposus and an outer ring, the annulus fibrosus.

*V̄t leuiori negocio, quæ
bic pertraclo, aſſequaris,
duas è thorace uertebras,
anteriori facie ex puerili
corpore depiclas habes. In
quibus 1 notat ſuperioris
uertebræ cartilaginem, ſui
corporis inferiorē appen
dicem, ipſumq̃ corpus in-
teruenientem, 2 eiuſdē uer
tebræ humiliorem appendicem, 3 cartilagineü ligamentum,
ſuperioris inferiorisq̃ uertebræ appēdices intercedēs, 4 ſu
periorem inferioris uertebræ appēdicem, 5 cartilaginem, di-
clam modò appendicem ſuæ uertebræ copulantem.*

FIG. 5. The structure of the intervertebral disc as drawn by Vesalius in 1543

Vesalius knew that the disc has a complex structure. He realized that the outermost layer is different from the inner material but he did not get the details absolutely right.

The nucleus consists of jelly-like material containing a few tangled fibres and many large molecules known as proteoglycans. The nucleus has the property of all gelatinous materials, namely that it can be squashed and then alters in shape but its total volume will remain constant. The nucleus is kept in shape by the outer annular ring and the vertebral end-plates above and below. This allows it to transmit the enormous loads that may be carried by the spine. It is the nature of the proteoglycans in the nucleus that they are constantly trying to suck in water and swell. This tendency is resisted by pressures produced by the weight of the body. When we sleep lying horizontally at night this swelling process is unimpeded. It is a fact that we are slightly taller when we first rise in the morning than at the end of the day. This process is carried to the extreme in spacemen who after several days of weightlessness may grow by a couple of inches. As their space suits are individually and very precisely designed this produced considerable difficulties and a lot of complaints from the spacemen before the cause was appreciated!

The annulus fibrosus which surrounds the nucleus has quite a different structure. It consists mainly of fibres of collagen. This is a fibrous protein which is uniquely designed for tensile or stretching strength. A collagen fibre is considerably stronger than a steel wire of the same dimensions. The collagen fibres of the annulus are attached around the edge of the vertebral end-plate and spiral obliquely upwards and downwards to the end-plates above and below. They cross over and interweave one another in a complex fashion so forming an extremely strong network that surrounds the nucleus. When vertical loads are placed on the spine the nucleus is squashed and slightly flattened and the annular ring will expand slightly, but nevertheless will not give way. Indeed the annulus is so strong that under extreme load it is the vertebral end-plates that will fracture rather than the annulus itself. This crisscross arrangement of annular fibres allows relatively easily the movements of bending forwards and backwards and to the side. However, twisting movements are more difficult. This is one of the reasons why back problems are more likely to arise with this type of activity.

At the back of the spine the vertebral arches are also joined to the arches above and below by the small facet joints. There is one joint on each side at each level so that connecting each pair of vertebrae are three joints: one between the vertebral bodies and two between the arches. The facet joints differ from the intervertebral disc in that they are synovial joints.

The opposing joint surfaces are covered by cartilage or gristle and are connected to each other by a fibrous capsule lined by a layer of tissue known as the synovial membrane. Within the joint is a lubricant known as synovial fluid which allows the joint surfaces to move against each other. This arrangement is very similar to that of the joints in the limbs, although the sizes and shapes of the various joints differ enormously. Any movement between a pair of vertebrae must involve all three joints; it is not possible for one of these joints to move to the exclusion of the others. It may seem trite to point this out but one often hears statements that one of these joints alone is stiff or that manipulation is applied to a single joint, ignoring the movements that must take place at the others.

The vertebrae are also joined to one another by a series of ligaments which ensheath the bodies and connect the arches. These ligaments are relatively flexible and yet have an important role in covering the bony and joint surfaces.

A pile of vertebrae one on top of the other is intrinsically unstable and one can readily imagine how bowing or slipping of the structure could occur. The spine is stabilized by very powerful muscles attached to the vertebrae, the pelvis, and the back of the chest wall. An interesting analogy is with the stays on a yacht which have a remarkably similar function in stiffening and stabilizing the mast. During any exertion these muscles contract so stiffening the spine and enabling it to bear the load.

The spinal cord emerges from the base of the brain and passes down through the vertebral canal behind the vertebral bodies and surrounded by the vertebral arches. During its passage downwards nerve roots separate off to emerge through the intervertebral foramina between the vertebral arches at every level. The spinal cord itself finally ends at about the junction between the first and second lumbar vertebrae (L1/2) and below that level there are only nerve roots in the vertebral canal. The roots emerge from the canal and pass on to their ultimate destinations, uniting and dividing in complex fashions to provide appropriate nerve supplies to all the structures of

FIG. 6. The stabilization of the spine by
muscles is remarkably similar to the stiffening of the mast of a yacht by the stays

the human body. The spine itself also has a nerve supply. Tiny
branches from the nerve roots will supply the ligaments
around the spine, the capsule (or surroundings of the facet
joints), the coat around the spinal cord, and the blood vessels
in the bone marrow. Surprisingly they do not occur in the
intervertebral disc. As damage to a nerve fibre is a prerequisite
for the sensation of pain, it is clear that disc disease alone will
be painless. It is only when a disc disorder produces damage
to other structures that pain may arise.

Another point about the nerve supply to the spine is that
the nerves from each level combine with one another in extremely complex fashion. This produces the phenomenon
known as cross-innervation which means that any nerve may
reflect abnormalities arising at several different levels. For

this reason it is often extremely difficult to localize the source of symptoms felt in the back. Pain felt at one site can be due to abnormalities at a quite different area. Considerable circumspection is required when trying to identify the source of the problem in the back pain subject.

The stresses on the spine

Because of the obvious practical problems it is remarkably difficult to gain objective information about exactly how the spine transmits load. Most of the data is derived from experiments conducted in Sweden on volunteers in whom fine needles were inserted into the intervertebral discs. The pressures developed during a variety of physical activities were recorded. As would be expected the lowest levels of pressure in the nucleus were found when lying down. High pressures developed when standing upright and even higher when carrying a heavy load. There were very high levels when sitting upright: the highest recorded were when sitting, bending forwards, and carrying a heavy load. In some people the total load on the disc was about 340 kg or about a third of a ton. The pressures developed could be related directly to posture, the load carried, and the contraction of the muscles stabilizing the spine. The posture of the back seems all-important. We know that a properly designed back-rest will relieve a lot of strain in the spine and in these experiments they found that a properly designed back rest or a good chair with a proper spinal support could significantly reduce the pressures within the disc during sitting.

Another way of getting at the problem is by measuring the pressures within the abdomen or tummy. At rest, the pressure in the abdomen is low. During exercise we forcibly contract the abdominal muscles and hold our breath, so contracting the diaphragm and increasing the pressure within the abdomen. Why do we do this? By increasing the pressure we convert the abdominal cavity into a high-pressure ball capable of carrying some of the body load. A pressurized ball, such as, say, a blown-up rugby football, will bear load and one could even sit on it without squashing it — that is, it will carry the weight of the body. On the other hand, if it is not blown up or has a leak and is under low pressure, by sitting on it one would flop on the ground — in other words low-pressure balls carry weight poorly. In a similar way, increasing the pressure in the abdomen allows a proportion of the body load to be transmitted through the abdomen and so relieves the spine to a certain extent. Weight-lifters do the same thing by putting on a strong leather cummerbund just prior to their lift.

The increase of the pressure within the abdomen is proportional to the total load on the trunk. This concept has been used to measure the stresses associated with various activities. Initially, measurements of the pressure within the abdomen were made using a balloon and a fine tube inserted through the anus and connected to an outside measuring instrument. Today there are sophisticated electronic measuring instruments that look like small pills and can be swallowed. Not only does the radio-pill measure the pressures but also it contains a tiny radio-transmitter and the signals can be picked up by a special radio receiver. The pills are safe and are eventually passed in the motions.

Most mechanical studies of the spine have been performed using post-mortem material. Clearly this information must be interpreted with caution as the dead spine is very different from that in life. In fact such studies have helped enormously in identifying the areas of potential weakness and where the stresses are most concentrated. They have shown that the back of the spine and particularly the arches carry a disproportionately large amount of the total body load and that this is increased by bending backwards. A careful examination of the spine will often reveal the evidence of damage produced by this means. This may take the form of small fractures of the bone or damage to the apophyseal joints.

The back of the disc is stressed more than the front of the disc. Although a single load is far more likely to damage the vertebral end-plates than the disc, nevertheless, it is possible that repetitive load could cause fatigue failure in the areas where the disc is most stressed. Indeed, these are just the places where disc damage is found.

In such a complex system with innumerable components, each serving important roles and interrelating with one another, it is hardly surprising that problems may arise. These may be due to abnormalities of development, damage due to excess forces, wear and tear damage due to repetitive use, and other problems. Subsequent chapters will deal with these various aspects and indicate the current limits of our understanding about them.

The causes of back pain

Failure to appreciate that every back pain is different and that there are many reasons why back pain occurs leads to much confusion. A form of treatment suitable for one problem may be useless for another so it is always necessary to try to determine the underlying cause. Back pain is a symptom just as being short of breath is a symptom. In thinking about how to treat breathlessness we would need to know whether the patient had bronchitis, asthma, tuberculosis, lung cancer, heart disease, or other problems. In the same way we should always try to establish the cause of the back pain, although admittedly this can be extremely difficult.

Pain may be felt in the back due to disease in the back itself or it may be a result of some internal abnormality but felt in the back. Gynaecological disorders may sometimes produce quite severe back symptoms and these are usually worse at the time of the menstrual periods.

There are a number of different broad groups of disorders of the spine that may lead to back pain. They include mechanical and structural problems as already mentioned; inflammation, which can be the result of infection, or other inflammatory disorders such as ankylosing spondylitis or rheumatoid arthritis; disorders of the structure of the bones of the spine; and tumours of various sorts that may occur in and around the back. Each of these groups includes a number of different disorders which will be described in this book.

The big problem is that there are many back sufferers in whom it is not possible to identify the cause of the symptoms. If such patients are seen by different physicians and surgeons, physiotherapists, osteopaths, and chiropractors, they may be given various diagnoses and the terms used are often quite different. A wide variety of different types of treatment may be offered. The patient may be perplexed and become more confused with every specialist he sees. The truth of the matter is that for many back problems, and particularly those that are relatively minor, it is not possible to identify the source of the problem. Although words such as fibrositis, adhesions, sacro-iliac strain, lumbo-sacral strain, etc. imply knowledge of what is actually wrong they have no scientific foundation and the various types of disorders have not been proven on examination of the spine by pathologists. My personal view is that with this degree of uncertainty it is better to be honest to the patient and to oneself and label the problem as 'non-specific back pain'. With newer diagnostic methods we are identifying with accuracy various problems within this group so that the number of patients in whom this uncertainty exists is slowly shrinking.

2

Back pain in society

The severity of backache ranges from minor niggles to excruciating pain but the problem as a whole is remarkably widespread. Any discussion on the subject almost inevitably brings out personal stories of individual attacks of back pain. In one survey conducted recently 21 per cent or over a fifth of the subjects questioned had suffered from back symptoms within the previous fortnight. Although many had relatively minor problems this must mean that most of us must suffer from back pain sooner or later. The back problem alone significantly interferes with enjoyment of life and with work in a large proportion of the population.

It is not enough simply to be aware that backache is common. We need to know the severity and extent of the problem and its relation to different types of work. This information is required not only for developing treatment services, but also to provide guidance with regard to occupational hazards and postural problems, on the premise that prevention is better than treatment. At first sight it would seem relatively easy to determine the severity of the back pain problem. However, there is a large number of complicating factors making such studies difficult and leading to a variety of ways of interpreting the results. It is worth explaining certain of these difficulties in some detail so that the conclusions drawn from such studies will be seen in a more realistic perspective.

Drawbacks of back pain surveys

Pain is an unpleasant emotional state felt in the mind but identified as arising in a part of the body. In other words it is a subjective sensation. The pain from, say, a boil occurs in the brain. Without the mind the pain would not exist, only

18

an area of swelling and inflammation. Pain is a defence mechanism designed to make the subject protect an injured part
from further damage. Sometimes, however, the mind can
make a mistake and feels pain when no cause exists or fails
to feel pain when there is good reason. There are reasons for
this which will be explained in Chapter 6. Because messages
reach the brain by a very complicated network of nerves
which connect with one another in various ways, the mind
may place the sensation as arising in the wrong place.

In other words back pain is a subjective sensation felt and
described by the sufferer and there is no objective means by
which the pain can be proven. The doctor must either believe
or disbelieve the patient's statement, whether or not there are
obvious things wrong with the back. In contrast a survey of,
say, tuberculosis of the lung can rely on hard evidence of the
disease shown by a chest X-ray.

To prove the presence of back pain it is not enough to
show that the back does not move properly or that an X-ray
is abnormal. Some people have a completely rigid spine which
is pain-free and others a back that is remarkably flexible and
yet are severely troubled by pain. The relationship between
symptoms of back pain and wear and tear changes on X-ray
is extremely poor.

This means that the only real test for back pain is whether
the subject can reliably describe it. Most people do not tell
lies when questioned on a topic such as this. However, we all
feel things differently and interpret pain sensations in different ways. There is enormous variation in the ways we respond
to particular stimuli and this must mean that the reporting of
pain sensations will differ greatly from person to person.

Different people feel pain to different extents. Some of us,
with a so-called high pain threshold, can tolerate a stimulus
such as pressure or a needle prick that another with a low
pain threshold may find extremely painful. These differences
between all of us depend upon a number of factors. They
may partly be racial or cultural, reflecting the normal and
acceptable forms of behaviour in our society. The ways in

19

which we feel pain may reflect other problems and anxieties which may not be very apparent. I know that if I am about to go on holiday I will ignore a bit of backache whereas if I am facing a difficult or unpleasant day it may seem very much worse.

As pain is a sensation which cannot be proven it is sometimes used as an excuse to avoid work or provide a day off. We have all heard of how the incidence of back pain seems to increase when there is an important football match or race meeting. Undoubtedly this sometimes happens but it is impossible to know how often back pain is falsely used in this way. Individual cases when they are known tend to stand out but my feeling is that the risk as a whole is somewhat overstated.

Many surveys of back pain will ask if the individual has ever suffered from this problem. There is a natural process in the mind to obliterate memories of painful events. The most extreme examples of this occur with severe accidents leading to unconsciousness. After recovery there may be complete loss of memory for the accident and for the events leading up to it. We often find that people will forget attacks of back pain in a similar way but to a much lesser extent. This poor recall of information about previous attacks of back pain can lead to serious underestimates of the frequency of this problem. As back pain usually develops in acute attacks between which the subject may be symptom-free, surveys analysing the frequency of this problem at any one time will provide only limited information and detailed and careful probing about previous episodes is required.

There are many different ways of performing back pain surveys. The information gathered will reflect the types of subjects studied and the information sought. This may seem obvious but serious errors have occurred by applying information gathered from a study of one group of subjects to a totally different group. To take obvious examples, a survey of back pain in children would provide very different answers from another in adults and a survey conducted in a coal-mining

PLATE 1. Computerized axial tomography *(upper)* and a CAT scan *(lower)* showing spinal stenosis (by courtesy of Professor I. Isherwood and Dr N. Antoun) (see Fig. 12).

PLATE 2. Obtaining an ultrasonic scan of the back (by courtesy of Mr R. W. Porter).

area would be very different from one in the stock-broker belt. We must ask whether the survey has been performed on all the people living in a particular area and whether it is a survey of the entire population, or people at work, and if the latter the type of work must be known.

The ways in which the surveys are performed also may influence the results. In industrial surveys the information that has been sought reflects the impact of back pain on work statistics, but this may give a very unreal view about the role of this problem in society at large. The numbers of working days lost due to back pain must be seen in relation to the type of job being performed. On the whole males do much heavier work than females but a greater prevalence of backache found in the male sex may not mean more back pain but simply that the males with perhaps the same degree of symptoms could not perform their more strenuous activities. Certain types of job cannot be performed by people with backache. If back sufferers avoided such work or rapidly left it, a survey would show a low incidence — an apparent contradiction.

Much of the information about days lost from work and the impact that the back pain problem makes upon society is derived from work records kept with varying degrees of accuracy. These results may be adequate for determining sick pay but not for the more detailed studies required for accurate statistical surveys.

The final problem is that in all the discussion in this chapter so far, I have treated back pain as a single entity. In fact we know that there are many different reasons why back pain may arise. They will be described in detail later on in this book. In determining the impact back pain makes on society it is expedient to lump them all together but this can lead to serious problems when comparing a short sharp bout of pain that is totally disabling for perhaps a few days with a less severe chronic problem that goes on for many years.

Despite all these difficulties much useful information has been gathered. This gives some guidance as to the risks of developing back pain and its relationship to particular types of occupation. The evidence between different surveys often conflicts to a certain extent but perhaps this is hardly surprising in view of the problems described.

Who gets back pain?

Pain in the back may develop at any age although it reaches its greatest frequency in adult life, being less frequent in younger people and also in old age. However, within the large group of disorders which may cause back pain there are certain conditions which are more likely to develop in certain age groups. For example, bursting of an intervertebral disc — the so-called 'slipped' disc — is most frequent at about 40–45 years. On the other hand ankylosing spondylitis usually appears in a much younger age group, commonly between 15 and 25 years. Although the frequency of back pain is relatively constant over a wide span of adult ages the proportion of people severely disabled by back pain virtually trebles in frequency in late middle age compared with young adults. It is disturbing that recently there has been an increasing incidence of backache reported in schoolchildren. It is not clear whether this is a real increase or simply that more attention is being paid to complaints that were previously ignored. An increase in the frequency of back pain in children is unwelcome but nevertheless it would also be of interest as it should be relatively easy to identify the factors responsible and therefore to develop long-term solutions.

A comparison of the incidence of back pain between the sexes produces surprising results. If the survey is conducted on the whole population it has been found that back pain occurs more frequently in women than in men. The reasons for this are not at all clear. It may be that women are more prone to spinal problems. There is a suggestion that childbearing might be responsible as we know that during pregnancy back pain may be produced because of the weight of the pregnant uterus and the increasing looseness of the spinal

22

ligaments. However, the greatest frequency in females occurs in those over 50 years old, making that explanation less likely, although it remains possible that the spine has been damaged to a certain extent during pregnancy leading to problems in later life. Another chauvinistic suggestion is that women feel pain more readily and complain more than men; in other words they have a lower pain threshold. This suggestion inevitably arouses indignation, probably with good reason.

However, if surveys are based on industry then there is a reversal of the situation and back pain appears more frequently in males. Each year there are 627 working days lost per 1000 males at work but only 347 per 1000 females. The reason for this is that males more commonly undertake heavier work. Not only may the job lead to a greater incidence of back pain but workers with back problems could probably continue in light work but not in heavy manual duties.

The risk of back pain is also related to one's body shape to a certain extent. There seems to be a higher incidence in those who are taller and heavier than the rest of us. As most of the body load is transmitted through the spine it seems likely that such people's backs undergo excessive stresses so that they are more readily damaged.

Although back pain usually is associated with stiffness of the spine there is an interesting group of back sufferers whose spine, and indeed all their joints, are more flexible than normal. Such people are probably born extremely supple and remain so throughout their lives but the excessive movements which occur may eventually lead to damage and back pain. They have been described as having the 'loose-back syndrome'. Ballet dancers are known to develop wear and tear forms of arthritis and it has been thought that this is simply due to them overtaxing their joints. However, we now find that ballet dancers have excessively mobile joints. In other words they have become good dancers because their joints are so supple; the joints have not been made supple by their dancing. This suppleness combined with the extremes of movement can eventually lead to premature wear and tear in the joints in the same way as the loose-back syndrome.

Back pain and life-style

A constant theme in the discussion of the back pain problem is the relationship between physical work and the development of back pain. There have been striking changes in the stresses associated with daily life during man's evolution. We all constantly perform lifting and carrying movements throughout the day. A recent calculation suggested that the pre-Neolithic hunter–gatherer man only performed about 50 lifts per day whereas twentieth-century man performs about 5000 lifts per day. The current rate is also much greater than in medieval times. Whether this alone or other aspects of modern society are responsible for the current incidence of the problem is hard to say but there is good evidence indicating that stresses can be important.

Surveys within industry show that the greatest incidence of loss of work due to back pain occurs in unskilled and older workers who are required to perform physically demanding jobs. The incidence of back pain in those employed in heavy industry is some five times that in light industry. However, the information available is not entirely consistent in that there is also a high incidence in those who perform sedentary work, particularly if they spend a lot of time driving motor vehicles. The incidence of back pain is higher in nurses (17 per cent) than in policemen (6 per cent): almost equal to that in heavy industry (22 per cent). At first sight this seems surprising but the stresses involved in lifting and turning heavy patients are probably equal to those in manual work. Policemen with backache may have to retire early because they lack the physical fitness required by the Force. Olympic weight-lifters do not develop more back pain than other workers but perhaps if they did they would cease to be suitable for such a competitive sport and therefore not be Olympic weight-lifters.

Back pain in society

The trouble with industrial surveys is that they usually cover the work force as a whole and within any industry there are numerous jobs, some of which may lead to particular forms of stress, but others may not. To take an obvious example, within the coal-mining industry, the coal face workers have quite different working conditions from those engaged in transporting coal, the underground electricians, the lift men, and the surface workers. Even at the coal face there are different types of work. Detailed analyses are necessary to identify the specific factors leading to the development of back problems in the individual job.

The greater incidence of back pain in those working in heavy industry has been mentioned. However, the term 'heavy industry' covers a multitude of working conditions and the precise problems causing back pain are still being identified. Perhaps it is the increased frequency of injuries occurring in those working in such an environment that is responsible. Acute injuries, twists, or sprains are frequently reported. If a person attempts to lift an unexpectedly heavy weight then the muscles stabilizing the spine fail to provide appropriate support and may lead to damage to the back and pain. Similarly an attempt to lift an unduly heavy object whilst stooping forwards is an important risk factor. A sudden twist, particularly whilst carrying a heavy object, can be responsible. We all have countless minor twists and strains which are rapidly forgotten but in some subjects they may lead to back problems.

Major injuries to the back are much more rare. They do occur, however, and can produce fractures of the spine. Fortunately these usually heal well but occasionally they may lead to persistent pain. Apart from sudden incidents of this type it does seem that those whose jobs make the greatest demands on their back are more likely to develop back pain. In particular stooping forwards and lifting a heavy object can lead to back problems. The incidence of back pain is much less in those who stand upright or walk about. There is a somewhat high incidence in those with desk jobs. It may be

25

that back sufferers preferentially choose such an occupation or possibly that continuous sitting leads to weakness of the muscles supporting the spine and therefore to back pain. Certainly poor seating can aggravate the situation. Sudden jarring and vibration movements have often been blamed for producing back pain. This may be why tractor drivers show a high incidence of this problem. There is a significantly increased frequency in those who are required to undertake a lot of driving in association with their work. Postmen who drive vans develop more back pain than those without driving commitments.

It therefore appears that there is a greater risk of back pain in those involved in heavy manual work. Of particular importance are jobs involving sudden and unexpected movements and prolonged stooping. Working in a poor posture, including sitting in unsuitable chairs, is a potent cause of back troubles. However, the information can be difficult to analyse and often the relationship between the back pain and work may be complicated by a compensation problem. If there is an identifiable cause that can be blamed on the job then the subject may expect some benefit. It is important to establish the facts of the matter but obviously this may colour the individual's response, either deliberately or subconsciously.

The incidence of back pain

Surveys of the incidence of backache show that it has been experienced by most of the population with very high rates in the older population. Over 4 per cent of people are likely to initiate a consultation from their general practitioner for back pain each year and it does seem that the frequency of consultations and of loss of work for this reason is gradually increasing. Less than a fifth of those who see their general practitioner for back pain are likely to be referred to a specialist, although, by reason of waiting list problems, many improve before being seen. One in thirty of these patients are likely to be admitted into hospital and of these only one in ten will have an operation. This means that less than 0.1 per cent of people seeing their general practitioner for back pain are likely eventually to have surgery.

The community burden

The global cost of the back pain problem to our society is important in indicating the importance of the problem and the need for extra resources to be directed to improving our current treatment facilities. Around 2 000 000 adults in Great Britain consult their general practitioners each year because of the development of back pain and this problem is the cause of 6.5 per cent of general practice consultations. The average GP will see 75 new back cases per year. In total there are 3.4 million consultations per year in general practice and 0.4 million patients are seen in hospital outpatient clinics. This means that 5 per cent of all new patients attending hospital for any reason are there because of their backs: 41 000 will be admitted and 3300 will undergo surgery.

In Great Britain in one year there were 750 000 spells of back pain with 19 200 000 working days lost; nearly 2 per cent of the population lose time from work each year because of back pain. At any one time some 10 000 people have been off work for six months or more and 4500 for two years or more.

Similar figures exist for the United States where over 7 000 000 Americans suffer from chronic low back pain and it affects 65–80 per cent at some time in their lives. More than one in three of Swiss people become unable to work at least once in their lives because of low back pain.

Economists love to quantify problems such as this in financial terms. A very crude estimate suggests the loss of output in Britain to be £220 000 000 per annum but this would not include invalidity benefits, the cost to the National Health Service of the general practitioners' time, the hospital services, and drug treatment, and it is impossible to provide any estimate of the value of the suffering experienced by the patient and his family.

Conclusions

The difficulties experienced in estimating the frequency of back pain have been described. Despite all these and much conflicting evidence it is very clear that back pain is one of the major problems in our society. It is possible to identify particular types of work associated with an increased risk of developing back pain but as yet the measures that have been taken have not led to a significant improvement in the incidence of the problem as a whole.

3

Discs—slipped or burst?

The phrase 'a slipped disc' is used very commonly and indeed at some time or other this diagnosis has been blamed for producing almost every form of acute back pain. There are two major errors in this. First of all discs do not and cannot slip, and secondly what does go wrong and may be called a 'slipped disc' is much less frequent than previously thought.

The correct term that should be used for patients with 'a slipped disc' is a 'prolapsed intervertebral disc'. What actually happens is that the disc bursts and fragments of the outer annulus fibrosus, together with some of the inner gelatinous nucleus pulposus, press on ligaments and nerves running close to the disc and produce pain. The term 'slipped disc' is not only wrong but also harmful as it leads to a false idea of what is happening and therefore of the likely outcome. The mental picture produced is of a flat biscuit-like structure that slips sideways or backwards between the bones of the spine. If the disc can slip out in such a fashion then it could equally well slip back again and all should be well. The truth of the matter is that the disc bursts so that it is permanently damaged. Once this has happened, that disc will never be normal again. Its resistance to further injury is considerably reduced and anyone who has had a burst intervertebral disc is always at risk of further episodes of acute pain. If I could make a plea it would be for the words 'a slipped disc' to disappear permanently.

Although backache has been suffered by man for countless millennia and the existence of intervertebral discs has been known for many centuries, it is only very recently that the two have been put together and that the idea of disc problems producing back pain has been accepted. Before that most mechanical types of backache were blamed on strains of the

29

various ligaments around the spine and problems with the small facet joints that lie towards the back of the vertebral column. The German pathologist, George Schmorl, had found small protrusions and leaks from the disc but did not think they were of any importance. The great advance was a study published in 1934 by two Boston surgeons, W. G. Mixter and J. S. Barr. They were treating a young man with acute back pain and for various reasons though that it might be due to a tumour in the spine. At operation they found a swelling at the back of the disc that was compressing a nerve root. After removal of the swelling the patient was cured. When the material removed at operation was examined under the microscope it was found to be lacking in cells. In contrast a tumour, and especially a cancer, would be full of cells that are dividing, so leading to growth. The material from the swelling looked very similar to that from a normal disc. When they compared the appearance with those found by Schmorl they realized that the whole problem was due to a prolapse or burst of the intervertebral disc. Further examination of other similar swellings removed at operation and in the pathology collection of the Massachusetts General Hospital in Boston showed that the majority were disc bursts.

The concept that the intervertebral disc can burst and so cause back pain and sciatica had enormous appeal to orthopaedic surgeons. The reason is that if back pain were blamed on strain of the ligaments or wear and tear of the spine not much could be done for it, whereas a burst would be amenable to surgical treatment. Something constructive could be offered. The swelling was removed, relieving the pressure on the damaged ligaments and nerves. Some of the disc substance was also taken away so that further leakage of material from the disc became unlikely. Following this remarkable discovery there was a tremendous surge of interest in the surgical treatment of back pain. At one time an operation was almost the standard procedure for the majority of back sufferers. The early results of surgery seemed good and for a while it seemed as if the back problem was solved. However, in recent years,

30

and in the light of experience, we now have a very much more cautious attitude to the use of operative treatment. The natural history of many back problems is of acute episodes of pain which sooner or later get better in most people. If surgery is undertaken too readily a successful result can be confused with the natural remission that would take place anyway. Operations, however small, always carry some risk and after back surgery there is a very definite incidence of further back problems that make one cautious in advising this form of treatment. Today, surgery is reserved for those in whom there is a very clear need, where damage that can be remedied has been identified with reasonable precision, and the patient has not responded to a period of more conservative treatment. In other words operations are the last resort for certain types of back pain rather than an immediate treatment as was the case a few years ago.

What goes wrong with the disc?

Although any disc in the entire spine can prolapse or burst, the most common ones to which this happens are the lowest two, that is between the fourth and fifth lumbar vertebrae and between the fifth lumbar and the top of the sacrum. Although the reasons for this are not entirely clear, the most likely explanation is that the stresses experienced by the spine are the greatest at these levels. Also the sacrum does not stand vertically but is tilted backwards, so producing a sharp curve in this region and giving a wedge shape to the discs. This wedge shape may concentrate the stresses in the back of the disc so making these lower lumbar discs particularly liable to damage.

Briefly, in a prolapse, the disc ruptures or bursts so that debris from the disc protrudes and can damage the surrounding structures. Most commonly these ruptures occur at the back of the disc but to one side or the other. These are known technically as the postero-lateral edges of the disc. Sometimes, however, the burst may occur directly backwards in the

FIG. 7. Backwards bursts of the discs between the fourth and fifth lumbar vertebrae, and between the fifth lumbar and first sacral vertebrae

FIG. 8. The disc bursts backwards and to one side pressing on the nerve root and other structures

32

midline and this is known as a central posterior prolapse. The direction the burst takes, together with the anatomical arrangement of surrounding structures, will determine the amount of damage that is produced and the type of symptoms that arise.

The backs of the vertebral bodies and the intervertebral discs are sheathed by tough fibrous material known as the posterior longitudinal ligament and this contains numerous tiny nerves. Interestingly the disc itself does not contain any nerves, so that disc damage alone could not produce back pain. It is likely that the acute pain felt in the back which occurs when the disc bursts is due to the damage of the posterior longitudinal ligament. Behind the ligament are the nerve roots which have separated from the spinal cord and are sweeping down through the vertebral canal to emerge through the openings between the vertebrae known as the intervertebral foramina. The material from the burst disc may breach the posterior longitudinal ligament and damage these nerve roots. A small burst may only damage one root whereas a larger one, particularly if it is towards the midline, may affect several. The damage to the nerve root will produce unpleasant sensations of pain, numbness, and tingling which are felt by the subject in the area that particular root supplies. In other words the pain will generally be felt in the lower limb. The damage may also interfere with the transmission of impulses down the nerve to motivate the muscles and this may cause weakness of particular movements. Some of the nerve roots also supply the bladder and the lower bowel. Damage here may lead to loss of control of passing urine and motions and sometimes to incontinence. When this occurs it is a major emergency and this is perhaps the only reason for immediate surgery for a prolapse. It is essential to relieve the pressure on these particular nerve roots as soon as possible in order to avoid permanent damage.

Why does the disc burst?

Use of the back, particularly heavy lifting, increases the pressure in the disc. An obvious explanation for what happens when the disc bursts would be that this pressure exceeds the strength of the outer annulus. Although this mechnism seems so simple, in fact there are important reasons why we now believe it is not the whole story.

Many episodes of disc rupture occur after quite trivial stresses – the sorts of stresses that we all undergo without noticing them. Some patients develop acute back pain after lifting a book, or twisting round, or perhaps mowing the lawn. It is difficult to believe that such forces are enough to produce a burst, but the changes in the spines of such people are the same as those occurring in other patients after damage by heavier loads.

For obvious reasons we are not able deliberately to subject human beings to loads to see what happens to the discs. However, although it seems a bit macabre, studies have been made of the spines of people who have died from accidents after sudden vertical forces on their spines. The most frequent cause of this is in people who receive fatal parachuting injuries when they land on their bottoms. The enormous forces experienced by their discs do not make the outer annulus of the intervertebral disc fail and do not produce the types of burst that are found in our patients. Examination of the spines have shown that if the forces are great enough the vertebral end-plates give way, but the annulus fibrosus remains intact.

Another approach to the problem has been to examine spines from people who have died from unrelated causes and subject them to forces and observe how the disc will fail when tested to the extreme. Such studies have been performed in several different ways but in general they show that the normal disc is so strong that it is the bony vertebral end-plate that gives way rather than the annulus fibrosus. Except under special circumstances force alone is not enough to produce a burst intevertebral disc. Further studies indicate that it is discs that were previously abnormal that will rupture in a way that resembles the burst disc occurring in life. The disc is already weakened by fissures, cracks, or degeneration and the stress experienced is merely the final event in making the disc burst.

The reasons for weakness or damage of the disc, placing it at risk of prolapse, are uncertain. One suggested cause is fatigue failure due to repetitive stresses similar to metal fatigue and failure after constant bending and straightening. The discs in different people differ in shape and in some the forces may become concentrated at a weak point, so gradually leading towards permanent damage.

These conclusions are clearly controversial because they have important medico-legal implications. If a person develops a rupture of an intervertebral disc while at work, it is likely that his disc was about to burst anyway as the disc was already weakened and damaged. The action that produced the rupture was merely the final incident making the burst occur, not the basic cause. There should be some doubt about whether legal claims are fully justifiable under such circumstances.

Symptoms

Although rupture of an intervertebral disc can occur at almost any age it is most frequent between 20 and 50 years and the peak incidence is between 40 and 45 years. It affects not only those involved in heavy manual work but also those who perform sedentary work who suddenly take unaccustomed exercise, for example office workers who spend their day at a desk and their evenings watching the television and who attack the garden or perform vigorous exercise at the weekend.

Some patients may have noticed warning symptoms over the few days prior to the prolapse. There may be aches and pains and stiffness in the back which herald the acute episode. The actual incident that precipitates the pain may be quite trivial, such as a sudden twist or bending forward to pick something up. The pain may strike immediately or it may develop gradually over a few minutes or a couple of hours. When it starts suddenly it is felt in the back and only later spreads down the lower limb. It may be so sudden that it feels like being struck and in Germany this has been called *hexenschuss*: a witch's blow. The pain may be so bad that the sufferer is unable to straighten up and finds himself stuck in the bent position and in great agony.

At first pain is felt in the lower back in the midline or to one or other side. This acute attack of pain is sometimes called 'acute lumbago'. After a while, maybe several hours, the pain spreads down the leg and may ease up in the back. This spreading into the leg occurs because the material that has burst out from the disc compresses and stretches the nerve root, and the area where pain is felt depends upon the particular nerve root involved. Commonly the pain is down the back of the thigh, the back or outside of the lower leg, and the outer edge and sometimes the top of the foot. There is also a sensation of numbness and tingling. Some people find it very difficult to identify the area where the pain is felt but find it easier to describe the site of tingling. The doctor will wish to know exactly where these abnormal sensations are felt as they help to tell him which particular nerve root is affected. These acute symptoms are made worse by straining, coughing, and sneezing, because these activities will raise the pressure within the vertebral canal adding slightly to the stress on the nerves.

The nerve roots that may be damaged by a burst join together in a complicated combination to form the sciatic nerve which runs down the back of the thigh to supply the lower limb. This is why the pain down the back of the leg is known as 'sciatica'. Sciatica can be agonizingly severe and may be made worse by movement and exercise.

It is rare for the nerves to the bladder and lower bowel to be affected but if they are there may be some loss of the normal sensations on passing urine and motions. Incontinence and soiling of the underclothes may occur. There may also be loss of ability to feel and a sensation of numbness in the saddle area. As already mentioned this is an emergency which requires immediate investigations and treatment.

Discs – slipped or burst?

The doctor's examination

The medical examination reveals various features which help the doctor to make the appropriate diagnosis. The patient is in pain and a simple look at the face will often indicate the severity of the problem. He may lie curled up or flat unwilling to move for fear of making things worse. The back itself may not be straight but may show a sharp twist, which is known technically as a 'scoliosis'. This occurs because the muscles on either side of the spine contract hard into spasm and pull the spine sideways. It is a reflex attempt by the body to twist the spine so as to relieve the pressure in the damaged area. It is possible to feel the muscles on either side of the spine and to detect the unequal muscle contraction. The doctor will watch the patient trying to move his back and will see that certain movements are virtually impossible whereas others may be relatively free. Bending forwards and to one side is most often limited whereas moving in the other directions is relatively little affected.

By careful palpation of the back it is sometimes possible to identify areas that are particularly tender and pressure may make the symptoms worse. This form of examination can give a crude idea of where the problem is but sometimes it may be inaccurate as the back pain and tenderness may be a little way from the actual site of the problem.

The lower limbs will be carefully examined to detect evidence of nerve damage. An important examination is the straight-leg-raising test. The patient lies on his back and the doctor raises the ankle as far as possible with the knee held out straight. In a normal person it is possible to bend the hip in this way between 70° and 90°. However in patients with sciatica straight leg raising makes the symptoms very much worse so that the movement becomes severely restricted. Some patients can tolerate only 10° of movement. Straight leg raising stretches the sciatic nerve and pulls on the nerve roots, stressing them that little bit more and therefore exacerbating the symptoms. Straight leg raising improves as

37

FIG. 9. The straight-leg-raising test

the back problem gets better and measurement of this movement is commonly used to follow the progress of the patient
with treatment.

The doctor will examine the power of various muscles in
the leg. He will test the reflexes, particularly the knee jerk
and the ankle jerk, and he will look for loss of ability to feel
sensations in the leg. With knowledge of the distribution of
the nerve roots he may then be able to work out which particular one has been damaged.

It is fortunate indeed that the vast majority of attacks of
back pain and sciatica due to a burst of an intervertebral disc
will get better spontaneously. With appropriate rest and treatment the symptoms gradually remit, often within a few days
but sometimes requiring a much longer period. The treatment
of acute back pain and sciatica will be described in Chapter 5.
If the symptoms fail to improve, then further and more detailed investigations will be required.

Investigations that may be performed

In the patient with a straightforward burst intervertebral disc
and acute low back pain and sciatica the diagnosis is obvious
and further tests may not be necessary. Blood tests and X-rays

need be performed only if there is some doubt about the diagnosis, or if the symptoms fail to get better and some further action is being considered. Briefly, all the blood tests should show normal results. Rupture of the disc does not affect the blood, so these tests are helpful only in checking whether some other condition may be present.

Ordinary X-rays of the back are equally uninformative. When we look at an X-ray we examine the shadows produced by structures interfering with a beam of X-rays falling on photographic film. Bones are relatively dense in contrast with soft tissues such as flesh so that a clear picture is seen and an abnormality in the bone, such as a fracture, is obvious. The intervertebral disc is made up of soft tissues which cast extremely faint shadows and cannot be seen in the spine because of the very dense surrounding bone of the vertebral column. For this reason it is not possible to see the bulge of the disc due to the burst. In patients with an acute prolapsed disc the X-ray may appear normal, other than perhaps showing the twist of the spine due to the sciatic scoliosis. However, the disc has lost some of its substance and further X-rays taken months or years later may show some loss of height of the disc and wear and tear changes of the surrounding vertebrae. This is one cause of the wear and tear changes, which are known as lumbar spondylosis and will be described in the next chapter.

More sophisticated techniques are available which are used to pick out the damaged disc and to show the burst. These methods are 'invasive', that is they involve special injections into the spine. They can be somewhat unpleasant and therefore they are reserved for those few patients in whom there are special problems, particularly those for whom an operation is being considered.

One technique involves injection of a special fluid that is opaque to X-rays directly into the vertebral canal. This fluid will occupy the space immediately behind the vertebral bodies and intervertebral discs. If there is any obstruction it will block the flow of this dye so that a space appears on the X-ray.

By this means it is possible to 'see' the burst accurately. Until very recently, the material that was injected was an oily fluid and the technique was known as myelography. Today, however, we use a new fluid that is watery rather than oily. This provides us with very much more better quality X-rays and much more detail of the nerve roots can be seen. The technique using this new fluid is known as radiculography.

There are some newer methods used in X-ray departments which are only available in special centres. One of the most promising is discography in which the radio-opaque fluid is injected directly into the intervertebral disc, using X-ray television to guide the direction of the needle. The examination is done under local anaesthetic. Not only does the method show if the disc is normal or not, but also injection of the disc that has burst and is responsible for the patient's symptoms will actually reproduce the problem during the time of the injection. In this way the disc that is at fault can be precisely identified.

4

Mechanical problems and backache

The spine is such a complex mechanical structure that it is hardly surprising that many things may go wrong. The most well known of these is the slipped disc, which should be called the burst or prolapsed disc. This has been dealt with at length in the previous chapter. However, there are many other mechanical problems that may arise in the spine and which actually occur much more frequently than a burst disc. In some of these the cause is obvious but in others it may not be clear and the symptoms are not severe enough to require the ultimate diagnostic test, namely surgery and examination of the offending part. In such cases the characteristics of the problem indicate some mechanical cause and usually some idea of its nature. It is not uncommon, however, for the experts to disagree on the precise fault as well as how it is best treated. Recent research combined with the use of advanced technology for diagnosis is helping to elucidate some of these very difficult problems.

Wear and tear in the spine

The spine of the young differs from that of the elderly. It is supple and flexible rather than stiff and rigid. The intervertebral disc is a springy cushion with a jelly-like centre but with age it becomes tough and fibrous with a reduction in its vertical height. The disc loses its ability to transmit forces in the optimum fashion and restricts the amount of movement allowed between the adjacent vertebrae. At the same time the bony surfaces above and below the discs, the vertebral endplates, also show wear and tear changes. The surfaces of the bone become thickened and a rim of bone develops around the edge of the disc. This is an automatic attempt by the body

41

FIG. 10. The vertebrae in a normal spine and in one
showing spondylosis with degenerative changes around
the intervertebral discs and in the facet joints

to splint the spine and to prevent further damage. These changes in and around the intervertebral discs are called spondylosis and in the low back are therefore known as lumbar spondylosis. Degenerative changes can also affect the small facet joints that lie behind and on either side of the vertebral canal. These joints are synovial joints — that is they contain a fluid-filled space with gliding cartilage surfaces and are similar in principal although not in detail to the joints in the limbs. Wear and tear in these joints is known as osteoarthritis. The cartilage becomes soft and can break up and its surface is worn away. The bone near the joint surfaces becomes thickened, especially around the rims of the facet joints, so adding to the splinting effect.

Although spondylosis and osteoarthritis are described separately they usually occur together so that it is difficult to distinguish the effects of one from the other. Wear and tear changes in the spine are remarkably common. They become much more frequent as we get older. This does not mean that the young are immune, however. The earliest changes may appear in the 20–30 year age group but at this age they are of course relatively mild. They become more frequent and severe with age so that by 60 years almost everybody has some wear and tear changes in the spine. They are so common that one must wonder if it is right to call them abnormal. If everyone develops spondylosis and osteoarthritis, surely that is 'normal' and the man whose spine remains as it was in his youth must be abnormal!

These wear and tear changes are diagnosed from X-rays of the back. It is relatively easy to see the spaces occupied by the discs on the X-rays but the facet joints are much more difficult. For this reason the diagnosis of osteoarthritis in the lumbar area is much less reliable than that of spondylosis. Even X-rays that show the changes in the discs are not as good as one might think. The disc itself is not opaque to X-rays and quite severe wear and tear in the disc substance may develop and yet the X-rays appear virtually normal. In my own studies of discs I found that the most trivial changes on X-rays could indicate gross damage to the disc.

43

Wear and tear does not affect all the discs in the lumbar region similarly. It is far more frequent in the lower two lumbar discs than in the upper three. This probably is due to the greater loads experienced by the low back and also the tilt backwards of the sacrum or tail bone so creating unequal stresses in various parts of the vertebrae and discs connected to it.

As these wear and tear changes occur so frequently we might infer that they are the cause of back pain, and the reason backache is so common. If every older person has lumbar spondylosis and osteoarthritis, we should all suffer from back pain sooner or later. As these changes are permanent, we should then have pain all the time. Fortunately this is far from the case but these points present the nub of the problem. Backache is common and these changes are common. However, in surveys in which the incidence of backache was compared with the frequency of wear and tear of the spine on X-ray, it was found that, although backache was more frequent in those with the worst X-rays, compared with those with normal or nearly normal X-rays the difference in frequency was remarkably small. Those with the grossest changes had only a 12 per cent higher incidence of back pain than those with the best X-rays. This must mean that in the majority of people wear and tear changes found by X-rays are not responsible for back pain.

This point has enormous significance but is often missed in ordinary clinical practice. A patient gets backache, an X-ray is taken and shows these wear and tear changes, and lo and behold the diagnosis is made. It is not nearly as easy as that. Many people with such changes do not have a back problem and if the symptoms are blamed on them other important causes of backache sooner or later will be missed. Simply finding these changes on X-rays is not enough. The clinical problems due to wear and tear of the spine are poorly defined; the symptoms and the findings on examination are not unique for this condition and may occur for other reasons. This adds to the confusion.

Mechanical problems and backache

This makes for scepticism about the value of X-rays of the back. Commonly patients with backache expect an X-ray to be taken and will feel dissatisfied with their doctor if one is not ordered. However, when the routine examination and blood test indicate nothing untoward, studies show that the X-ray does not make any useful contribution to the diagnosis or treatment. All X-irradiation is harmful, the amount of risk depending on the dose of X-rays. Taking an X-ray of the low back requires quite a high dose with a small but definite risk to the ovaries in women and the testes in men. It is possible to protect these organs to a great extent but it is far better to avoid unnecessary X-rays.

Commonly, symptoms due to lumbar spondylosis and osteoarthritis develop as one gets older and produce aching and stiffness in the low back. The symptoms are often intermittent with good and bad periods and sometimes the back can feel quite normal between attacks. Pain is felt in the back but may spread into the buttock and sometimes down the thighs. Posture seems all-important in producing symptoms. Bending forwards, and particularly lifting heavy weights, sitting in a poor chair, and sleeping on a soft mattress all make things worse. It is usually possible to find a position of comfort and most patients find that standing upright or sitting with the back properly supported will provide relief. These points are dealt with in more detail in Chapters 5 and 8. The symptoms in the back are made worse by exercise and on the whole are easier after rest, although some patients sieze up and take a minute or two to get going after prolonged inactivity.

The most obvious feature of the back with lumbar spondylosis and osteoarthritis is loss of its ability to move. There is stiffness on bending forwards and backwards and attempts at these movements can make the pain worse. Sometimes bending or twisting the back sideways may also be restricted although generally these movements are relatively unaffected. There is one form of degenerative change in the back which may be so widespread that the whole spine becomes stiff and then all movement is lost. Interestingly though this is not usually a painful condition. Movement at a damaged joint causes pain. When the spine is completely rigid there is no pain.

Some back sufferers can identify the part of their back which is the most painful and careful feeling may show that it is tender. This palpation technique can indicate the particular region of the spine which is responsible for the symptoms. However, it is not always accurate because of the complex ways in which the nerves supplying the spine itself combine with one another. The symptoms and tenderness can be at an area quite different from that actually responsible for the problem.

All this indicates that the whole concept of wear and tear in the spine producing backache is unsatisfactory. Undoubtedly it is responsible in some people but its presence can be misleading in others.

Fractures

If one breaks a bone in the arm or leg it is extremely painful. The fracture is rested in a sling or in a plaster-of-Paris cast and gradually it will heal. New bone grows across the break and connects the two ends, eventually to form a solid structure again. At the same time the severe pain during the fracture improves. If the two broken bone ends are not properly held but are free to move against each other severe pain will be felt and healing will be delayed. With appropriate splinting the improvement in symptoms is much more rapid and healing enhanced.

Precisely the same type of problem can affect the back. A major accident can cause a fracture of the spine. Most often there is crushing of one of the vertebral bodies. There will be very severe pain in the back and the subject will be scared to move for fear of making the pain worse. At its worst these fractures may damage the spinal cord or nerve roots. Paraplegia, or paralysis of the legs, following an accident to the

46

spine, develops in this way. With rest the fractured vertebra will gradually heal, although the back never regains its former shape, and the back pain will usually get better. The evidence of the injury can be seen on X-rays for life.

Such gross fractures as these are obvious and fortunately are uncommon. We now know however that much smaller fractures may occur and actually are quite frequent. They are difficult to recognize on X-rays and that is why the diagnosis is so often missed. Small fractures may occur in the vertebral arches at the back of the spinal column. This is because these parts of the spine normally transmit a very large proportion of the total force and this is enormously increased by bending the spine backwards. Examination of this part of the spine by X-rays is very difficult. The detail is not clear and tiny fractures of this sort are easily missed. Only special X-ray techniques provide the clarity of detail required and even by using the most up-to-date methods it is likely that many cases are missed. I have seen patients with acute back pain that developed following some excessive exertion. The special X-rays showed the tiny fracture. After a few days' rest the pain improved; subsequent X-rays showed the healing of the fracture site. There must be many people with acute back pain for this reason in whom the symptoms are blamed on damage to the ligaments or other structures or on wear and tear of the spine.

Bone is not a uniform material but consists of a thick outer coat containing within it a meshwork of filaments known as trabeculae. These trabeculae are very thin threads of bone and form the inner framework of the whole structure. Between them lie the blood-forming cells of the bone marrow. Fractures of these tiny trabeculae are quite common. They are so small that they are known as micro-fractures. Often they occur close to the vertebral end-plates where stresses are concentrated. I believe that overloading the spine can produce a micro-fracture and severe pain just as any other fracture would. With rest the fracture site heals and the pain gets better. Unfortunately, the X-ray techniques available today will not provide enough detail of these trabeculae, so we have no method of diagnosing these micro-fractures in life. Advances may make this possible in the future.

Vertebral slips

The vertebrae sit one on top of another, forming a column. Normally these vertebrae remain in place but sometimes one vertebra may slip forwards or backwards on the one below. A forward slip is known as a spondylolisthesis and a backward slip as a retrolisthesis. There are two main ways in which the spine becomes unstable in this way. One is a break in the bony arch at the back of the vertebra so that the stabilizing action of the elements at the back of the spine is lost. Until recently it was thought that these breaks occurred because the arch had not developed properly during childhood. However, we now believe that most occur due to a fracture following injury. This fails to heal, so leaving the spine unstable. The second mechanism is wear and tear of the spine, which can also allow the vertebrae to slip. With spondylosis, excessive movement appears between the vertebrae and the slip develops.

The patient with a vertebral slip suffers from back pain because of damage to the spinal ligaments. The nerve roots become stretched at the site of the slip so that problems develop in the lower limbs. Naturally symptoms are made worse by moving the back. The diagnosis is made from the X-rays.

Increased mobility

Some of us are more supple than others. It is this characteristic which distinguishes good dancers and sportsmen from the rest of us. At first sight this increased mobility would seem to be an advantage but in certain conditions it can be carried to an extreme and then be a real handicap.

There are certain medical disorders of looseness of the

supporting tissues of the body. The principal ones are known as Ehlers–Danlos and Marfan's syndromes. People with these disorders may have such loose joints that they can twist and bend them in ways not available to the rest of us. Certain forms of these conditions produce the 'India-rubber men' that we see in the circus. This looseness of the tissues can affect other structures besides the joints and sometimes lead to internal damage. In most people being loose-jointed or 'double-jointed' does not carry any risk of internal problems. However, such people are at risk of damaging their joints very easily and eventually may develop premature wear and tear changes.

Ballet dancers have very supple joints. Girls become ballet dancers because they are born with joints more supple than normal rather than the other way round, although practising exercises which make the joints more supple obviously helps. Even joints not used in exercises and dancing are found to be much more flexible than normal in ballet dancers, who have a greater risk of wear and tear damage to their joints than the rest of us. It seems that the excessive stresses to which they subject their joints is responsible. The same sort of problem can also occur in footballers. A good footballer has more supple joints than normal so that he can twist and turn with a fluency that is beyond most people. Those footballers who are more supple are at greater risk of damaging their joints in the long run.

Similar problems occur in the back. Some of us have excessively flexible spines. A useful test is to try and touch your toes with your legs straight. Most of us can almost or just about get there but the hypermobile person will not only get there but can even place the palms of his hands flat on the floor. This excessive movement can lead to premature wear and tear damage in the spine and recurrent back pain, a problem which has been called the 'loose-back syndrome'. Back pain develops, particularly on movement. If the physician fails to appreciate the basis of the problem he can be very surprised how mobile the back is with such severe symptoms.

normal

hypermobile

FIG. 11. Normal and hypermobile backs

Mechanical problems and backache

Abnormal mobility can develop in another way. If for any reason one section of the spine is stiff there may be excessive movement above or below this segment in order to compensate for it. We often find that this excessive movement in one localized region leads to severe degenerative changes and symptoms at that level. The pain is produced not by the stiff segment itself but by the compensating excessive movement that is associated with it. Observation of the back can sometimes show which areas move normally and which abnormally but generally the diagnosis is made from X-rays. In order to diagnose this problem properly the X-rays are sometimes taken with the spine both bent forwards and backwards, to show the full range of movements.

Narrowing of the vertebral canal

As explained previously, the nerve roots pass down through the vertebral canal and emerge through the openings at the sides of the spinal column known as the intervertebral foramina. Canals differ considerably in size and shape between different people. In most of us the canal is quite large but in some it is relatively small, so that the nerve roots are much more tightly packed. The trefoil canal is an abnormality in shape of special importance. The nerve root about to leave the canal passes through a very shallow recess which is only just large enough to accommodate it: space is very tight. Any protrusion into it will inevitably injure the nerve root, whereas if there were an open canal it would merely push the root aside without causing damage. This problem of narrowing of the vertebral canal is known as spinal stenosis. It is quite common, occurring in about 15 per cent of the population. Usually the spine has just grown that way but sometimes the bony thickening developing around the disc borders and facet joints in degenerative disease or for other reasons can reduce the canal dimensions.

Anyone with spinal stenosis is at special risk of developing back pain from an intrusion into the canal space. In practice

51

FIG. 12. Spine canal shapes — normal and spinal stenosis

PLATE 3. Modern traction.

PLATE 4. Isometric exercises.
Upper: To strengthen the abdominal muscles. *Lower:* To strengthen the spinal muscles.

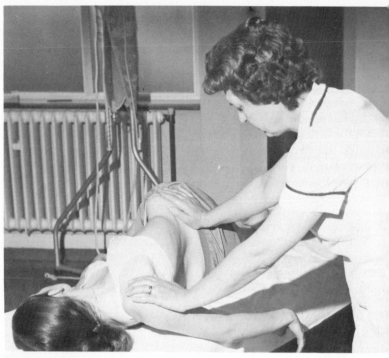
PLATE 5. Maitland's mobilization of the spine.

we now know that people who develop sciatica due to a burst intervertebral disc have smaller canals than normal. They have been put at risk because of their canal size and if they had had a larger canal, the burst disc would probably not lead to serious back problems.

There is a characteristic pattern of symptoms associated with narrowing of the canal. The patient develops low back pain with numbness, tingling, and painful cramps in the lower limb. These occur on exercise and may develop after walking several hundred yards; sometimes they are sufficiently severe to force the patient to stop and rest. After five or ten minutes the pain gradually gets better. It occurs in this way because exercise increases the blood flow within the vertebral canal and this alone may squash the tightly packed nerve roots that little bit extra necessary to produce pain. This pattern of symptoms is often confused with 'intermittent claudication' — painful cramps developing in the calf due to an obstructed blood supply to the leg. In claudication the pain symptoms develop on walking and are relieved by rest in a similar but not identical fashion. When there is narrowing of the vertebral canal, the blood supply to the legs, and in particular the pulses in the feet, are normal.

The physical dimensions of the vertebral canal are slightly larger when the spine is bent forwards than when it is bent backwards. Because of this the pain may be relieved or prevented by flexing forwards. This accounts for the curious phenomenon experienced by those patients who find that walking produces the symptoms whereas they are able to cycle for long periods without any pain. They walk with their spines upright but cycle with them bent forwards.

Sometimes however, the clinical problem is not as clear cut as this and we now know that narrowing of the canal increases the risk of other types of back pain. It is important to make the diagnosis as it can be quite easy to reduce the pressure on the nerve roots by an operation. Unfortunately it is difficult to determine the size and shape of the canal by ordinary tests. X-rays taken from front to back or from side to side will give only very limited information. What is needed is a vertical view of the vertebral canal, but of course it is not possible to get such a view in life using conventional X-ray techniques. For this reason there has been considerable interest in the newer technologies which have been adapted to solving this particular problem.

The first such method is known as radiographic stereo-plotting. It has developed from a technique in use by land surveyors to show the contours of the ground. They take a series of photographs from an aeroplane and look at pairs of these photographs through binoculars to obtain a three-dimensional view of the land. With extremely complicated optical equipment it is possible to plot out the contours of the ground with considerable accuracy. The same technique was used by the spacecraft orbiting the moon to find flat areas on which to land. In radiographic stereo-plotting a pair of X-rays are taken with an alteration in the position of the X-ray beam between exposures. These are viewed through binoculars and it is possible to see the shape of the vertebral canal as a solid structure in three dimensions. By complicated optics using a computer the canal dimensions are measured. Although this method is both effective and helpful it is remark-ably time-consuming and also tiring for the observer who has to look through the binoculars for considerable periods in order to make the measurements. It is therefore only useful as a research tool and it seems unlikely that it will ever come into day-to-day use.

The latest method involving X-rays is the computerized axial tomographic scan or CAT scan for short (Plate 1). This method was invented by Geoffrey Hounsfield, an engineer working for EMI in Hayes, Middlesex. He shared the Nobel Prize for this development as it has revolutionized many X-ray techniques and is particularly useful for brain disorders. The method involves passing a beam of X-rays through the body and recording the transmitted signal on the other side. The beam and the recorder are rotated around the part being studied and the information received is processed in a com-

puter. By making an extraordinary number of complex calculations the computer will build up and reconstruct a picture
of a horizontal section across the human body. This gives the
vertical view that is lacking using conventional X-rays. With
this technique applied to the human spine it is now possible
to see the size and shape of the vertebral canal and recognize
those patients in whom it is abnormal. In practice this method
is rapid and effective. It is unfortunate that the apparatus is
incredibly expensive and this makes it unlikely that CAT-
scanning will become generally available for back problems in
the foreseeable future.

A new technique that shows great promise does not use X-
rays but instead an ultrasonic beam. This is a beam of sound
waves of such high frequency that they are not audible to
man. When this beam passes through tissues it bounces back
at hard bony surfaces to produce an echo which can be measured electronically. By recording the time it takes for the
echo to return the distance that the beam has travelled can be
calculated (Plate 2). This beam is applied to the spine by
placing the transmitter on the back just to one side of the
midline and shining the beam towards the vertebral bodies. It
is then possible to make measurements of the depth of the
spinal canal. The apparatus is already available in most hospitals; it is commonly used in pregnancy to determine the position of the baby in the abdomen, and for other purposes. It
is not expensive and the test is relatively easy to perform as
well as not carrying the risks of X-rays. However, only time
will tell how valuable a method it is.

Other abnormalities of development of the spine

No two spines are identical and the range of differences can
be enormous. Normally five lumbar vertebrae sit on top of
the sacrum. On occasions there may only be four with the
last lumbar vertebra actually joined into the sacral bone. In
others there may be six lumbar vertebrae, the first part of the
sacrum being free and appearing as an additional lumbar

vertebra. There are other abnormalities in which the spine appears inadequately formed or of somewhat abnormal shape. These and other variations are common and in general it can be stated that they do not produce any back pain. It is important to appreciate this and not to blame backache on them too readily. The only time such abnormalities of development can give rise to trouble is if they alter the mobility of associated parts of the spine and lead to premature wear and tear changes.

The various types of non-specific back pain

The difficulties in deciding on the true diagnosis in this very large group of back problems has already been mentioned. There are many people with constant or recurrent backache, perhaps exacerbated by stooping and sometimes with acute episodes but who are relatively well between attacks of pain. The characteristics of the symptoms and findings on examination may suggest a mechanical cause but the diagnostic terms that are used are often very unsatisfactory. It is particularly this group that produces much of the confusion in our understanding of the whole back problem. Some of these patients have X-ray changes indicating wear and tear of the spine but it has already been mentioned how difficult it is to ascertain the true significance of such features. The ultimate test, examination of the tissues, is rarely if ever possible as an operation is hardly ever required.

With the doubts that exist about the true diagnosis it is better to label these problems as 'non-specific back pain'. This term indicates back pain of uncertain cause but with any serious disorder excluded. This is an honest appraisal of our understanding and avoids deluding both the patient and the doctor that the cause of the pain is properly understood. Within the whole group of non-specific back pains, we can now pick out various entities with varying degrees of certainty or uncertainty but so often the problem is confusing with the same patient being given a variety of diagnoses by different physicians.

Mechanical problems and backache

If the ankle is twisted suddenly the ligaments are over-stretched and become swollen and very painful. In other words we have a sprained ankle. In the damaged ligament there may be bleeding and torn fibres. There is some inflammation which helps to repair the injury but also adds to the swelling. That ligament may occasionally be permanently damaged, or overstretched so that the support for the ankle is weak and the ankle can easily be injured again.

The same sort of problem may affect the back. A sudden movement of the spine may overstretch and strain the ligaments around the vertebral column in just the same way as at the ankle. The damaged ligaments are painful and yet the ranges of movements of the back are normal or even increased. The continued movement leads to further ligament strains.

Those double-jointed people described earlier may meet the same sort of problem. With their excessive flexibility they may stress the spine to such extremes that damage to a ligament takes place.

Ligaments can be strained in another way. To take a simple example, if one rests in a chair with the feet up on a stool, aching and stiffness may develop in the back of the knee. This is due to stretching of the ligaments behind the knee joint. Similarly if one sits or stands in a poor posture then the various ligaments connecting the vertebrae may be over-stretched and this will lead to an aching pain felt in the back. Most of us experience this if we sit for a long time in a soft armchair without any back support. When we get up and move about the aching and stiffness gradually disappear.

In people with strained ligaments the spine usually retains a good range of movement — if anything, greater than normal. Carefully feeling the back may show an area of tenderness, particularly if a ligament near the surface is damaged. Pressure at this point may reproduce the symptoms.

Following damage to the ligament there is a repair process in which fibrous tissue is formed. This is a scar that stiffens the ligament so that in the end movements become more limited than before the accident. An area of fibrous stiffening is called an adhesion and may be painful because it is stretched during relatively normal movements. The persistent stiffness seen in the back after injury is due to adhesions around the joints of the spine. Sometimes adhesions form around nerve roots so that back movements pull on the nerves and produce pain in the back and lower limbs. The most severe examples of adhesions can occur in those patients who have worn a lumbo-sacral corset for a long time after a back injury. They have kept their spines very still and avoided movements and the end-result is this severe stiffness. Any attempt at movement produces severe pain because of stretching of the adhesions. I call this condition a 'stuck back'.

Fibrositis is a common complaint, and yet no one really understands what it is. The term 'fibrositis' refers to pains felt in localized areas across the shoulders or in the back. There are very tender and painful spots or nodules in the muscles and the symptoms become much worse with any exercise. Careful feeling sometimes indicates that the muscle in that area is contracting continuously or, in other words, in spasm. The reason why this happens is not clear but the result is that the blood supply in that area is poor and the waste materials formed during normal muscle contraction are not carried away. This may contribute to the pain. Usually these painful areas will respond to a local injection.

Sometimes the pain is felt in one or other of the two sacro-iliac joints that connect the sacrum or tail bone with the rest of the pelvis. These two joints are based low down in the back with one on each side. They are very complicated and irregular joints and usually only allow a very limited amount of movement. There is a common inflammatory disease occurring in the sacro-iliac joints, known as ankylosing spondylitis, which will be described in Chapter 9. However, it is also possible to develop pain in these joints because of mechanical damage. Pregnancy is the most common cause. In the female pelvis it is normal for the various ligaments to become much looser at about the time of childbirth so that the pelvis can enlarge and the baby be delivered without damage. During the later stages of pregnancy backache is common and this is partly due to the looseness of the various ligaments allowing the pelvic joints to widen combined with the extra strain on the back produced by the weight of the pregnant womb. Once childbirth is completed the ligaments gradually return to their normal condition and the looseness of the sacro-iliac and other joints disappears. In some women, however, the joints may not return to exactly their previous fit and the ligaments may remain overstretched. These sacro-iliac joints can be very painful. The pain is felt in the low back in one or other sacro-iliac joint and is made worse by bending and twisting movements. Mothers have to do a lot of bending, particularly when looking after a new-born child, and consequently often have backache and tenderness in the area of these joints.

There are many other types of backache that do not fit readily into these groups. The nature of the symptoms and the examination findings will indicate no serious illness but suggest that there is some form of mechanical problem. It is valuable to be able to reassure the patient that there is nothing seriously amiss but at the same time we must acknowledge that the current state of affairs is still unsatisfactory. With the greater insight into non-specific back pain that we have today, and by using newer diagnostic methods, we are gradually learning to identify the underlying problems. There have been real advances but there is still a long way to go.

5

Physical methods of treatment

Introduction

Back pain can develop for so many different reasons that it is
no small wonder that there is such a wide variety of forms of
treatment. The problems of defining the precise cause of the
pain are reflected in the often difficult decisions about the
best types of treatment. What is suitable for one back sufferer
may be quite useless for another. Some people will respond
rapidly and effectively to one type of treatment whereas
others with superficially similar problems fail to obtain any
benefit. As we get better at establishing the precise causes of
the back pain we become able to offer more definite advice
and help. However, in many cases the types of treatment
used depend predominantly on the severity and nature of the
symptoms, rather than being specifically directed at the underlying problem. Clearly the long-term future lies in acquiring a
better understanding of the spine and its problems.

This chapter describes the physical treatment of patients
with the various mechanical types of back pain. The control
of pain, as opposed to treatment of the back, is described in
Chapter 6, and injections and operations in Chapter 7. The
spinal problems associated with other disorders such as
ankylosing spondylitis, Paget's disease, tumours, and so on
are considered separately under their appropriate headings.

Many patients with back problems suffer from acute episodes of pain and disability with little problem in between. It
is usually relatively straightforward to deal with these acute
attacks but continuous or recurrent problems can be much
more difficult.

Physical methods of treatment

Beds and bed-rest

For the patient with very severe low back pain, particularly if he has a burst intervertebral disc, there is one golden rule that if obeyed will almost always clear the symptoms within a reasonably short period of time. The subject must lie flat in bed until the symptoms are better. There is a great temptation for many sufferers with such pain to try to continue as normal and pay only lip-service to proper bed-rest. I have seen many patients who have struggled on like this for months without relief, or with symptoms that came and went with periods when things seem to be getting better followed by sudden and depressing relapses. When put to bed in the way described below the symptoms usually will clear within a few days or couple of weeks. It is for this reason that people with severe back pain and sciatica are often admitted to hospital. There are many temptations to get up and around at home, and complete bed-rest can be hard to achieve. The eagle eye of the hospital ward sister can work wonders!

The phrase 'complete bed-rest' means that the patient must stay in bed lying flat virtually all day long. Some doctors even insist that they lie flat whilst eating meals and washing, and that they must use a bed pan. In my own view it is not essential to be quite so strict and I allow my patients up to wash and to go to the toilet. This is principally because I feel that the strain on the back is much less if one gets up briefly than if one perches precariously on a bed pan or struggles to wash whilst lying flat. However, they must be careful and avoid any movements that produce pain.

This period of rest in bed continues until the pain is better. Generally the pain in the back and down the leg will start to improve within a few days and the important test showing the severity of the burst, namely the angle of straight leg raising, gradually increases. Sometimes improvement may take two or three weeks. If the patient is no better at the end of this period then some other form of treatment may be required.

Back pain: the facts

Not all beds are the same. Following a night in a poor bed many of us will wake in the morning with aching and stiffness in the back. This problem is far worse for the back pain sufferer and if put to bed it is essential that the bed conditions are right. The big problem is that many beds are soft and sag under the weight of the body. The softness of the beds is often equated with quality but this is not so. A good bed will have a soft surface which is resilient and does not sag. If the bed is too soft the weight of the body will make the bed give, so that the spine lies in a curved position. Lying on one's side makes the back curve sideways and lying on one's back makes it bend forwards. Both these positions can make the symptoms much worse.

How can one obtain the ideal bed, and what should one do if suddenly confronted with the need to provide complete bed-rest for the back sufferer? The simplest answer is to place a board under the mattress and on top of the base of the bed. This board will support the mattress and prevent sagging without making the bed uncomfortable. The board should be the full length of the bed and at least as wide as the subject. It should be rigid enough not to bend under the body weight. Three-quarter-inch blockboard seems a very good material for this purpose. Smaller boards are available and also folding boards that may be taken by back sufferers with them if they have to sleep away from home. Although they are helpful these folding boards cost a lot more and are not quite as rigid as the type of board first described. For people who sleep in a double bed it is often a good idea for the board to be placed under both partners. Sleeping with a board is remarkably comfortable and even the non-sufferer may be pleasantly surprised once he has tried it. Because double beds are so large it may be necessary to have two separate boards side by side underneath the mattress.

An alternative way of providing support to the back during the night is to place the mattress directly on the floor. It can sometimes be a bit draughty but as far as the back is concerned it does just as well. Some hardy people prefer to sleep

62

Physical methods of treatment

FIG. 13. Beds. *Upper:* The sag in a poor bed. *Centre:* The support from a properly sprung bed. *Lower:* A board under the mattress

directly on the floor. The hardness of the surface and the cold do not seem to worry them. For most back sufferers, however, this is not necessary.

The ideal solution may be to buy a bed which will give appropriate support. This is where the quality of the bed comes in. A cheap bed contains few springs which are widely spaced so that it readily sags under a load. This can usually be recognized simply by sitting on the edge of the bed when the 'give' is all too obvious. In better-quality products there are many more springs which are set closer together. There is much firmer and smoother support, preventing sagging. Unfortunately quality has its price and the cost of the better beds can be much higher than of the cheaper products. Any reputable shop selling beds will provide information about the firmness of their products and about their construction.

'Orthopaedic' beds are widely advertised as being suitable for the back pain patient. In this context the word 'orthopaedic' means that the bed is particularly firm. The term 'ortho' means straight and 'paedic' refers to children so that the original use of the word orthopaedic referred to the type of surgeon who corrected the deformities of crippled children. It then came to refer to surgeons who dealt with all disorders of the bones and joints but it is not at all clear why this adjective should be attached to the description of a bed when no surgery is involved. The adjective orthopaedic is often used to justify an enormous increase in the cost of the bed compared with other similar products which are obtainable at much more reasonable prices.

When buying a bed it is important to choose one that is appropriate and comfortable for the person who will use it. Lie on the bed in the shop for a few minutes and see that it feels comfortable and that there is no sagging. However, a bed that is too firm and too hard can be uncomfortable. There is no better way than trying it out for oneself. There is no general rule about which bed is best. A large, heavy person may need a different type of bed from a small, light person. In some cases one person in a couple needs a firm

64

bed but the other prefers a relatively soft bed, and there are combination beds that may be zipped together to give this type of arrangement.

The back sufferer lying in bed must lie flat. This means that only one pillow is allowed. More than that will twist the neck and the spine and can stretch the nerves and ligaments in the back, aggravating the symptoms.

The patient with severe back pain will be confined to bed. However, this description of the sleeping arrangements applies to any back sufferer. Many people with backache have some of the worst symptoms at night or first thing in the morning. Lying flat with a firm bed will usually make an enormous difference to these problems.

This advice about beds applies not only to people with back pain but may be used as a guide for anybody seeking to purchase a bed. Even people without backache will find that a firm bed with proper support is much more comfortable than one that sags too readily. Calculations show that the average person spends 23 years of his life in bed. It must be worthwhile getting one that is comfortable. In other countries people are accustomed to different types of beds. In the United States they are usually much firmer than in Britain and American visitors often complain of discomfort and back problems due to the soft beds when visiting here.

Why does bed-rest help?

Very severe attacks of back pain and sciatica are usually due to damage in the spine and often a burst intervertebral disc. There is not only the mechanical problem produced by the injury but also some inflammation of the damaged tissues. The inflamed tissues are swollen and produce pain. Every time the back moves these swollen tissues are rubbed, producing more pain and more inflammation. In this way keeping active never allows the injured part of the body to heal. A period of complete bed-rest lets the inflammation settle and hastens the process of healing. Again, a rather crude comparison can be drawn with a boil. If it is continually rubbed it will take a long time to get better but left alone it will clear up rapidly.

Curvature of the spine stretches the nerves and the ligaments. When the spine is straight there is the least strain on them. This is why it is important to avoid sagging.

As the pain clears up the patient can gradually start moving again. At first things should be taken very cautiously but within a week or two the subject should be able to get back to reasonable activity. However, he must always be careful to avoid stressing his back. Advice on posture and the correct ways to bend and lift will be given later.

The recovery period

We are dealing with back pain due to mechanical damage, and clearly any undue strain of the back can make this worse. It is very important to make sure that no undue stress arises, particularly during the healing phase after an acute attack of pain. It is only too easy to damage the back again and lose the benefit from a long and boring period of bed rest. Getting out of bed should be done gradually and carefully, using the arms to push oneself up sideways and avoiding bending the back as much as possible. When standing one should not perform sudden movements, particularly if they involve bending and twisting. Any movement that produces pain is bad and should be avoided. When first getting up it may be helpful to hold on to a rail or some other object in order to get support.

Avoid lifting altogether if possible. If it is really necessary the load must not be too heavy and it is better to divide it into two or more parts rather than lift a single heavy object. Lifts from the floor should always be done by bending at the knees with one foot behind and the other at the side of the object keeping the spine straight rather than flexing forwards. This is described in detail in Chapter 8.

When lifting an object, take up the strain gradually rather than suddenly. A sudden jolt to the back may be enough to cause another attack of back pain. When carrying any weight it should be held as close to the body as possible. This is because holding it further away produces a much greater stress on the spine than when it is held close. Above all do not carry any object that is too heavy.

When sitting down the type of chair is all-important. Chairs for back sufferers, or indeed for any of us, are dealt with in detail in Chapter 8. Here suffice it to say that the chair must be of the appropriate height and should provide support in the small of the back. Low armchairs with soft padding might superficially look comfortable but they can make the back problem much worse. An upright chair with a built-in lumbar support or a small pillow placed in the hollow of the back is better and very much more comfortable.

Instruction on the care of the back is all-important. If you know how to protect the back it is relatively easy to avoid stressful situations and to prevent recurrence of the problem. This process of instruction has been carried to an extreme in Sweden where they have now developed 'back schools'. The whole treatment programme revolves around teaching the back sufferer about the structure of his back, what may go wrong, and how to protect against further damage. There are a series of class lessons and at the end of the course the patient takes an examination which will not only tell whether he has understood all that has gone on, but also act as a revision exercise, going over much of the material covered in the course. The Swedish doctors and physiotherapists who run the back school feel that the end-results are as good as those obtained using other types of treatment. Their work looks promising; and understanding of the problem can only help – after all that is the reason why this book has been written.

Traction

It is a constant source of amazement to me that traction as a treatment for back pain has been used for many centuries and persists in principle relatively unchanged to this day.

Moreover, despite the frequency with which it is practised, we do not know how traction works, and indeed there is still doubt about whether it works at all.

A Paries excauatus.
B Columna querna quadrata pannis ftrata.
C Habena pectori circundata.
D Laqueus fupra genu & talos.
E Habena ilibus circumiecta.
F Piftilla ad caput & pedes.
G Affer è tilia.

FIG. 14. Traction combined with pressure on the spine as recommended by Hippocrates. By courtesy of the Wellcome Trustees

Hippocrates was a physician in ancient Greece and his writings are still relevant to many medical problems today. He treated back pain by traction in which the patient lay prone on a board known as a scamnum. Ropes were tied to the upper and lower parts of the body and a winch tightened, so stretching the spine. This treatment was often accompanied by some form of manipulation. Sometimes the manipulator walked barefoot over the stretched spine. Barefoot manipulation, often by female manipulators, is still practised today and is said by some to be remarkably relaxing, particularly if performed under appropriate circumstances!

Another technique used in ancient Greece was to hang the poor back sufferer upside-down by his ankles from an upright ladder. The ladder was then shaken vigorously and the pain was said to get better. Of course if the pain got worse there was little the patient could do about it in such extenuating circumstances.

A related technique is still practised by some people as a form of 'do-it-yourself' traction. The subject stands against a door with his hands hooked over the upper edge and then gradually relaxes and bends the knees until the feet are lifted off the floor. It is all-important to do this slowly and carefully as otherwise it may not only make the back pain worse, but also pull the door off its hinges. The spine should be twisted carefully from side to side and the weight gradually transferred to the feet as soon as the hands begin to tire.

Traction is sometimes used for people in acute back pain when confined to bed. Bandages are tied around each leg and a rope is bound into each bandage. The two ropes from each leg run over pulleys positioned at the foot of the bed and weights of a few pounds are attached to each. In order to stop the traction pulling the subject down the bed, the foot of the bed is raised a few inches so that the body will counter-balance the weights. The stretching force applied is very mild as it is kept on for long periods. As such it is doubtful whether such force actually does anything to the spine. More likely it is a very effective means of making sure the subject rests properly as it is not possible to get out of bed without un-doing the traction.

With intermittent traction, much more powerful forces are applied. This is performed under the close supervision of a physiotherapist to make sure no damage is done. The subject is strapped with a harness around the lower chest and pelvis and lies on a special traction couch. The two halves of the body are pulled apart so that the low back is stretched with forces of 30–60 kg (70–130 lb) (Plate 3). The precise arrange-ment varies with the back problem, the type of couch, and the physiotherapist giving the treatment. The couch is posi-tioned so that the subject is comfortable and the stretching is arranged so as to avoid making the symptoms worse. The pull may be either continuous for several minutes or gentle repetitive rhythmic pulses of stretching and relaxing. Speculation has it that rhythmic traction improves the circulation to the spine.

It is not at all clear what traction does to the back and how it may relieve back pain. The original idea was that the tiny facet joints in the back of the spine had become displaced and that pulling on the spine would bring them back into alignment. However, examination of the spine produces no evidence to support this. Another theory was that stretching the spine would suck the 'slipped disc' back into its original place in a similar fashion to the way we can suck toothpaste back into a half empty tube by stretching the tube. However, we now know that discs do not slip but burst and it is difficult to see how traction on the spine could suck a burst disc back again. It could be that pulling on muscles that have contracted in spasm may gradually make them relax and so relieve the pain.

There is a novel method of applying traction to the low back which does not require the subject to lie in a bed or on a special couch. The apparatus consists of a firm girdle around the pelvis and another around the lower chest connected by vertical ratchets on each side. By lengthening these ratchets the low back is gradually stretched. There is also a special pad which presses on the low back to provide lumbar support. The patient can walk, sit, or stand whilst wearing this apparatus. It remains to be seen whether the results are as good as or an improvement on those obtained by more conventional means.

It is difficult to assess the value of traction as it is commonly combined with other forms of treatment. Most patients with acute back pain and sciatica confined to bed will get better within a few days or a couple of weeks. It is difficult to say whether traction actually hastens this process or simply makes the bed-rest more effective. When given on an intermittent basis it is often combined with heat, exercises, or manipulation. Most patients slowly improve after a short period of regular treatment. In a careful study conducted at

Physical methods of treatment

St. Thomas's Hospital in London, patients were given intermittent traction either with the full force for 30 minutes per day, five days per week for three weeks, or else a very light traction given in a similar fashion. Those receiving the full force did slightly better than those receiving only minimal traction but analysis of the statistics did not indicate that the extra improvement was of real significance. So it remains an open question whether traction either by itself or in combination with other forms of treatment is of real value.

Heat and cold

We all know how comforting warmth can be for backache. A warm bath or a hot water bottle can be remarkably relaxing. Those prone to backache often wear thermal underwear such as an angora wool vest. In many countries the national dress seems to reflect this and the wide woollen cummerbunds found in many peasant costumes could well have developed on this basis. In Britain, Doll's flannel was traditionally worn and seems to have had the same purpose.

On the other hand, draughts are notorious for producing backache. It is not at all clear why this should be. One theory is that exposure to cold makes blood vessels contract, reducing the blood supply to the tissues in and around the spine and causing pain. Another suggestion is simply that lying in a draught often means that one is keeping still in an uncomfortable position for a long period. Either or both of these may be true. All we know is that in some unknown way lying in a chill can exacerbate back pain.

This sort of experience led to the use of heat to relieve backache. The simplest method is to apply a hot water bottle or expose the back to a radiant fire. Many people do this for themselves and they must always be extremely careful not to overdo things and burn their back. It is often easy to see that patients have been applying radiant heat to the back as it produces a curious and persistent mottling of the skin which can last for a long time after stopping the treatment.

Back pain: the facts

Heat is frequently used by physiotherapists as part of a programme for back pain. They do not believe that the heat alters the underlying problem or makes any difference to the long-term outcome. However, it is effective at relieving the symptoms at the time it is given and they use it as an adjunct to other types of treatment. Heat is given to the stiff and painful back as a preliminary to exercise or manipulation.

Heat can be applied directly to the back using electric heating pads. This heats the skin but is not very effective at heating the deeper tissues. Both infra-red and short-wave diathermy are able to penetrate the skin and therefore seem more effective. Infra-red is a form of heat radiation similar to light waves but of a wavelength beyond the extremes of the visual spectrum. All hot objects radiate infra-red waves but some materials are much more effective radiators than others. Radiant heat lamps are very efficient and the infra-red radiation is applied to the back in a careful fashion and a measured amount of heat given. The short-wave diathermy machine is very different. Electric currents circulate in a special coil placed over the back. They induce electric currents beneath the surface of the skin and generate heat within the body tissues. The short-wave diathermy apparatus is extremely expensive. There is now real doubt about whether it has any advantage over simpler methods of applying heat. In some recent studies in which the temperature was actually measured beneath the surface of the skin, it was found that the temperature rise is very much less than previously thought. Moreover, there are special problems with short-wave diathermy as it can induce very strong currents if there are any metallic objects beneath the coil of the machine. Short-wave is now used much less frequently than it was a few years ago.

Massage

Massage, or the rhythmical application of pressure by the hands, can be remarkably comforting for people with acutely painful backs. A skilled masseuse can relax tight knotted muscles and dissipate much of the pain. Although such treatment sounds remarkably pleasant and comforting, unfortunately in the long run it does not actually alter the course of the back pain. It does nothing to the underlying problem but merely alleviates the symptoms for the time that it is given. Massage may work by altering the perception of pain rather than by improving the damaged tissues. This will be described in Chapter 6.

Massage seems more helpful for people with acutely strained backs than those with long-standing chronic back problems. It is sometimes given in combination with other types of treatment, making manipulation and other procedures less painful. This type of treatment is sometimes used for sportsmen with a minor injury when skilled massage combined with heat and exercises may get them back to full activity more quickly.

It therefore seems that massage has a minor but nevertheless helpful part to play in treating some back problems. It is unfortunate that the technique has become synonymous in the popular press with various types of sexual activity and the masseuse with a therapist of a not strictly medical kind. This has led to loss of the skills possessed by practitioners of this technique. Although they seem of limited value nevertheless they can be helpful under appropriate circumstances.

Various types of liniments are sometimes used. They are slightly irritant ointments rubbed into the skin over the painful part. Reddening of the skin results partly due to the chemicals within the liniment but also due to the actual rubbing itself and indeed this is another form of massage. The relief of pain seems to be due to a combination of both these factors.

Exercises

At first sight exercises seem the obvious way to cure the stiff and painful back. Stiffness should improve and painful joints and ligaments eased back into normal use. The keep-fit experts extoll the virtues of exercises and mobility in the belief that physical fitness can prevent and cure most ills. However, what may seem obvious is not necessarily true. Even the fittest athletes may be struck down by acute attacks of back pain and those lazy members of society who avoid virtually all forms of physical activity may escape without any significant back problems.

Do regular exercises prevent back pain?

This question is not as easy to answer as it seems because, although on the whole fit people get less back problems than those who do not take regular exercise, it may simply be that those with backache are not as good at sport or keep-fit classes and therefore turn their attentions elsewhere. The inference to be drawn is not that performing athletics prevents the development of back pain but that people with backache do not become great athletes. Future research should help to solve this conundrum.

What about the value of exercises for a person who has had or who is recovering from an episode of back pain? Exercise treatments are often prescribed yet the evidence about their value remains in some doubt. There are various types of exercise programmes and they will be considered separately.

In general, exercise treatment is avoided if the pain is very severe or if there is a lot of spasm of the muscles, as forced movements can make the problem worse. There is much debate over which type of exercise is best. A golden rule is that if a movement exacerbates the problem then it should be avoided. After all if there is some damage to the spine and a particular way of moving the back aggravates the symptoms then surely it makes sense to avoid that movement. The best rule when exercising the back is to keep within the limits that the symptoms themselves impose. If severe pain develops at the time, or if so much exercise is performed that the back is very painful afterwards, then too much has been done.

There are two main reasons why exercises are performed.

Physical methods of treatment

The first is to stretch joints in the spine so that their movements are restored to the normal range. The second is to improve the strength of the muscles so that less strain is carried by the bones and joints. Both of these aims are of value under the right circumstances.

Types of exercises

In mobilizing exercises, the principal aim is to improve the movements of the back by bending the spine in all directions in an effort to overcome the stiffness in the various joints. The subject stands upright with the hands above the head and bends forward to touch the toes and then upright and arches backwards as far as possible. Sideways bending is performed by standing upright with the arms by the side and then sliding first one hand down one thigh and then the other way, from side to side. Twisting movements of the back are performed in clockwise and anti-clockwise directions. Although this type of treatment is used by many therapists, in general I do not favour it as it is extremely vigorous and often seems to do more harm than good. The weak back can be further damaged by these extreme movements and the whole problem made worse. Although some individuals seem to get better careful studies have shown that in general these mobilizing exercises have no real value.

There are only two problems for which I think these mobilizing exercises are right. The first is a quite different condition, namely ankylosing spondylitis, which will be described in Chapter 9. The second is for people who have had an attack of back pain and then have worn a corset for a very long time thereafter. If the spine is not allowed to move properly for such a long period, adhesions may develop between the joints so that the spine becomes extremely stiff and all movements very painful. At this stage movements in all directions are severely limited and any attempt at bending stretches the adhesions and produces pain. I call this a 'stuck back' and I think it is as much due to the past treatment as to the original back injury. For such patients I think that mobilizing exercises can be very helpful. They stretch the adhesions and gradually improve the movements of the back. Of course, as the back has been stuck for such a long time mobilization can be a very painful process and pain-relieving tablets are necessary. If the subject persists with the exercises it may be possible to get the back almost to normal. It is important that this treatment is carefully supervised to make sure no harm is being done.

In flexion exercises the emphasis is on forward bending. Not only are these performed standing upright as previously described, but also lying flat on the ground with the hands above the head and then forcibly sitting up and bending forwards to touch the toes with the legs outstretched. These exercises are extremely vigorous. Although they may be suitable for athletes who aim to keep themselves in the peak of condition, generally they are not right for the back sufferer. The bending movements can squeeze the discs and stretch the ligaments. A burst disc that has healed can easily burst again under these circumstances. Back sufferers should not perform these forcible flexion exercises.

Similar doubts arise about extension exercises, in which the subject stands upright and forcibly arches backwards. The bones in the back of the spine normally carry an excessive proportion of the load compared with other parts of the vertebral column. Arching backwards increases this and can add to damage in the tiny facet joints in the back of the spine. Studies comparing these extension exercises with other types of treatment have shown that they are of no value, and for some people they may make things worse.

The type of treatment that is of real value is known as 'isometric' exercises. These are aimed at building up the muscles of the back and also of the wall of the abdomen or tummy. Strengthening the spine muscles provides much better control of back movements, and enables the patient to lift and perform other activities with less stress on the bones. Improvement of the power of the muscles in the abdomen will increase the pressure that can be produced in the tummy and therefore will relieve the back of a greater proportion of its load. Isometric exercises will produce these benefits without stressing the spine itself and therefore are very helpful.

The word 'isometric' comes from 'iso' which means equal and 'metric' which refers to length. Isometric contraction of a muscle means that the muscles contract without altering their length. Pulling on a rigid object is an example of an isometric contraction. If the object moves then the contraction is no longer isometric. The principle of isometric exercises is applied to the spine by making various muscles contract but with minimal movements of the back itself (Plate 4).

The muscles of the abdomen can be strengthened by lying flat on the floor, pointing the toes and raising the head to look at them. Another method is to lie flat, raise both legs straight in the air, and then lower them slowly to the ground. These are very effective exercises for the tummy muscles and do not stress the spine at all. The back muscles can also be strengthened by lying prone or face downwards with the arms by the sides and then lifting first the head and shoulders and then the legs alternately. Each position should be held for a few seconds and then relaxed. Each movement is performed half a dozen times. It is only necessary to lift the head and shoulders and the legs off the ground and the back should not be arched excessively. If pain is produced the exercise should be done more gently. However, all exercises are tailored for the individual and his problem, and the physician and physiotherapist will advise on what is appropriate.

In general, exercise treatment is directed at strengthening muscles rather than improving the movements. It is only too easy to make the back worse and any exercise or movement that produces pain should be avoided.

Manipulation

Of all the problems associated with back pain it is the question of manipulation that gives rise to the greatest controversy. A wide variety of different manipulative techniques is practised both by medical practitioners and lay persons. The different methods are taught in different schools often with no agreement as to when manipulation is indicated, what is being treated, what actually happens during the manipulation, or the short- and long-term results of treatment. Moreover, personal views are often expressed vehemently but without any scientific foundation.

We have all heard of patients severely disabled by back pain who obtained immediate relief following a manipulation. Nevertheless the overall value of these procedures remains in doubt. Some studies have been performed to determine whether manipulation works. Despite these investigations a solid case in favour of manipulation remains unproven. My own studies of these techniques will be described. A recent working group convened by the Department of Health and Social Security to investigate the whole back problem emphasized these doubts and pointed the need for further research.

The mechanical basis for the majority of back problems suggests the possibility of a mechanical solution. If, as osteopaths suggest, there is a spinal 'lesion' or 'derangement' which consists of a slightly dislocated or subluxed joint or some loss of mobility, then a manipulation may put things right. But it is not as easy as that. Many back problems arise from a burst of the disc. No amount of manipulation can repair a burst. A damaged ligament cannot be repaired by manipulation. So the controversy persists, although to the patient what matters is whether the technique works rather than why or how it is done.

The origins of manipulation

The word 'manipulate' when applied to the spine refers specifically to manual pressure on the back in an attempt to

78

remedy defects. In biblical times physicians believed that back pain could arise because the bones were out of alignment and that manipulation could line them up again. The Greek physician Galen described methods of combining pressure on the spine with traction techniques in an effort to restore alignment. Nevertheless manipulation did not find favour with the medical profession in succeeding centuries and was largely ignored until quite recently.

Until about a century ago medicine and surgery were different professions. The physician believed in the prescription of elegant mixtures of medicines which commonly had little or no therapeutic action, but were usually impressively coloured and unpleasant to take. The surgeon was there to operate and performed such procedures as amputations, opening of the abdomen for various types of stones, and stitching wounds. The patient with a strained joint would often go to the bone-setter who would try to put things right by giving the joint a wrench or a twist. The physicians and surgeons of the day looked down on bone-setting as a crude, unprofessional, working-class type of treatment and not to be considered in the sophisticated society in which they mixed. Nevertheless some bone-setters developed reputations of being able to treat bad backs and enquiring minds began to examine the value of these procedures.

Bone-setting was a very crude form of manipulation. Little attempt was made to identify what had gone wrong and why. Rather all patients received the same type of treatment, for better or worse. The bone-setters were practical people, not theorists, and did not worry too much about whether they actually did what they thought they were doing but whether they got good results. They believed they could realign displaced joints by breaking down the adhesions, holding them out of alignment, and then reducing them back into the appropriate position with a satisfying 'plop'.

Perhaps the most famous bone-setter was Herbert Barker who practised in Manchester and London in the early part of the twentieth century. His work was condemned by the medical profession and his case was made worse by being sued by a youth whose tuberculous leg he had treated and which later was amputated. Nevertheless his reputation grew. He developed a reputation for treating back pain for which eventually he was knighted. Whether his results would stand up to critical modern analysis will never be known.

Osteopathy

The bone-setters were practical men who practised their art according to rules which neglected whys and wherefores, and only sought results. Osteopathy, on the other hand, grew up with a theoretical basis. Although osteopathic techniques may well be helpful, many of the original ideas were extremely controversial and subsequently have been discarded.

The founder of osteopathy, Andrew Taylor Still, was an American physician in the nineteenth century. (He is not to be confused with George Frederick Still of the Hospital for Sick Children, Great Ormond Street in London, who first described arthritis in children.) A. T. Still believed that the spinal cord and the nerves, particularly in the neck, controlled the blood flow in the limbs and elsewhere. Disorders of the spine, such as a strain or a partial dislocation that he called a 'subluxation', could disturb the blood flow and produce various types of symptoms. By manipulating the neck he believed it possible to improve the blood flow and cure all sorts of symptoms and diseases. Osteopaths believed in the osteopathic 'lesion' – a disorder of the intervertebral joints which could produce not only pain in that area but also many other problems including heart and lung disease and various abdominal upsets. The extravagance of the osteopaths' claims were unacceptable to the medical profession and led the whole subject into disrepute.

Today most osteopaths believe firmly that their form of treatment may help various types of spinal disorder and the pain that is produced by pressure on nerves and other structures, but that the excessive claims of past years are best forgotten.

Physical methods of treatment

The osteopath will examine the spine for what he calls a 'lesion' or derangement. Carefully feeling this area reveals some loss of the normal mobility in an intervertebral joint. We do not know the pathological basis for this osteopathic lesion — if indeed there is one. Many different things can go wrong in the spine and in life it is often difficult if not impossible to prove what has happened to produce the impaired mobility about which the osteopaths speak. The osteopaths themselves are in doubt and suggest a malalignment of the vertebrae, adhesions between the joints in mobile segments, and other explanations.

Osteopaths carry the technique of palpation to a fine art and use a variety of terms to describe the changes in the various spinal segments. These findings are entirely subjective and it is very doubtful whether they would stand up to comparison by two different experts examining the same patient.

Once the area believed responsible for the problem is identified the osteopath will manipulate the spine. When patients are seen repeatedly the preliminary examination is always performed first so that the manipulative technique can be modified according to the patient's progress.

The treatment involves relaxing the muscles around the affected part by careful stretching and manipulation, moving the affected joints carefully and repeatedly until free, and following this with a 'high-velocity thrust' using lever techniques on the pelvis and other parts of the body. The patient is usually positioned on his side and with a twist to the trunk so that other joints in the back are believed to be locked and only those that require treatment are free. The 'thrust' may sometimes produce a tearing noise and a click. It is uncertain what produces these sounds. Some osteopaths think that they represent the tearing of adhesions between joints and therefore regard them as a good thing. In fact we do not know what is happening and there does seem some potential risk if unknown tissues are being damaged internally.

Of course what counts in the end is whether the treatment works, and it is all too easy to adopt a rough and ready approach and say that if any practitioner can make the back better then he should get on with it. While this is true the statement does contain a big 'if'. Although many backs do improve after an osteopathic manipulation it remains to be proven that the treatment itself was responsible for the improvement and that it has made any long-term difference. What is certain is that any manipulative therapy should only be given by someone who is properly trained. Although robust, the spine is a very complicated structure containing many delicate nerves and tiny blood vessels. Unskilled or wrong treatment can do a lot of harm.

Does osteopathy work? If it can be proven helpful then all else will be forgiven. The techniques would be adopted by the medical profession and particularly by those concerned with treating pain. Before too long the osteopaths might find themselves out of business. The problem is that the techniques of osteopathic manipulation have never been submitted to the type of scientific enquiry that is routine for all other branches of medicine.

Attacks of back pain do not normally persist indefinitely but come and go with acute episodes that may last a few hours, days, or weeks, but will almost always partially or totally clear up until the next bout develops. If treatment is given during an acute attack the chances are that the attack will get better anyway and it is uncertain whether the treatment itself was responsible for the improvement. Anecdotal stories of people with persistent back problems who get better immediately after osteopathic manipulation are quite common but equally I have known patients who have described similar improvement after forms of treatment which I know are of no value. These included the use of a deep heat machine applied to the back but with the current turned down so low as to be totally ineffective. This was applied in a trial in comparison with another form of treatment to be described later. Nevertheless some patients do get better and it seems likely that osteopathic manipulation can have some immediate benefit.

Physical methods of treatment

The long-term benefits from this type of treatment are even more doubtful. If osteopathy is useful it probably hastens an improvement likely to occur anyway, but does not make any real difference in the long run, nor does it protect against future attacks of back pain.

Are there any harmful effects from osteopathy? In the first place back pain can be due to causes other than the type of mechanical problem in which the manipulators specialize. Osteopathic manipulation for ankylosing spondylitis, cancers in the back, and other conditions can do considerable harm. It is always important to be certain that no other condition is present before undergoing such treatment. An osteopath who has not received a broad medical training may miss these other disorders and manipulate when it is contra-indicated. I have seen a patient who had a small tumour in the spine that was responsible for pain; manipulation produced severe damage to the spinal cord and paralysis of the limbs.

The force of manipulation can be quite strong. It is extremely rare that bones are fractured but ligaments can be damaged and some patients can be made worse rather than better by the twisting that is performed.

So there is still some real doubt about osteopathy. Many patients see osteopaths and are pleased with the results. Others are disappointed or even find themselves worse after the treatment. I would advise that such treatment be given by a medically qualified osteopath. Even under such circumstances it remains uncertain what is being treated, what the treatment actually does to the spine, whether it is of real immediate value and whether there is any long-term benefit. Careful studies should be undertaken in which patients whom the osteopaths consider suitable for such treatment are either given osteopathic manipulation or some other innocuous form of treatment and their progress followed over succeeding days, weeks, and months to determine the true value of the method. By analysing the information it should be possible to elucidate these points and if the treatment is helpful to try to find out precisely the types of problem for which it is most suitable.

Back pain: the facts

Chiropractic

At the same time as osteopathy developed, another school concentrating on spinal manipulation grew up and was called chiropractic. According to legend the system was developed by D. D. Palmer, who treated a case of deafness with a sharp thrust to the neck. Chiropractic is based on the belief that poor alignment or partial dislocation of the bones of the neck impinge upon nerves and can be responsible for many types of illness. Manipulation of the neck is thought to correct these mechanical faults and restore body health. Chiropractors believed that their form of manipulation was the treatment not only for spinal pain but also asthma, high blood pressure, migraine, and many other diseases. It is hardly surprising that such claims led to tremendous controversy and considerable doubts about the value of the technique and about its practitioners.

Today most chiropractors concentrate on mechanical problems in the spine and try to forget the exaggerated claims of yesteryear. They believe that joints may either be fixed or displaced beyond their normal ranges of movement, producing various structural and functional changes not only at that site but also in remote tissues, by damaging the nerves. They believe that a poor posture can also be responsible for the symptoms, and that these structural defects can be corrected by manipulation, so making the patient better.

The techniques employed by chiropractors differ from those of osteopaths, who concentrate on twisting the spine by using the shoulders and pelvis as levers. The chiropractor manipulates the vertebrae themselves. The thrust is a rapid but not very powerful force applied directly to the vertebrae. The chiropractor concentrates on determining which type of thrust is appropriate and delivering it with precision.

Once again we have the difficulty of establishing how much value lies in the technique. Although many individual patients seem to do well either immediately or after several treatments there are many others in whom it does not work or who even become worse. The course of back pain is often unpredictable. The analysis of the particular structure at fault often varies between chiropractors. The types of thrust used may differ. The method and skill of application depend very much on the individual practitioner. It is hardly surprising that it is almost impossible to know quite how good chiropractic is.

The status of osteopaths and chiropractors

There has been an interesting divergence in the establishment of osteopathy and chiropractic in Britain and in the United States of America. In Britain there are some osteopaths who are medically qualified. They usually trained as doctors first, became interested in back pain as a problem, and then learned the techniques and practice of osteopathy. However, the majority of osteopaths are not medically qualified but have undergone training in a school of osteopathy. There are considerably fewer chiropractors than osteopaths. In general they are not medically trained but qualified from a college of chiropractors.

In contrast, in the United States the differences between osteopaths and chiropractors have tended to disappear. Many use whichever technique from either profession seems most appropriate for the particular patient. Their training has become increasingly similar to that of medical students and their practice very much like that of general practitioners in this country. They may use drugs and sign medical certificates and indeed some may undertake very little in the way of manipulation. In other words many osteopaths and chiropractors have become another form of doctor. In ordinary clinical care one may be unable to distinguish whether the practitioner had a formal medical training or learned his medicine by these alternative methods. One can readily imagine a new breed of manipulators developing in the United States as the osteopath and chiropractors increasingly become aligned to conventional medicine.

85

Back pain: the facts

Manipulation by physicians, surgeons, and physiotherapists

Although most doctors do not receive formal training in their student days in the techniques of manipulation, some will learn how to do so and use it for treating back pain patients. There is much controversy about the various forms manipulation can take and about their values. Some doctors may learn osteopathic methods and even attend a special school training physicians in these techniques. Others will learn by postgraduate courses or by working with more experienced colleagues. Although treatment by both medically qualified and lay manipulators can be similar, the advantage of the former is a broad understanding of medicine with the result that other conditions that can masquerade as back pain will not be missed. If one goes to a lay manipulator then almost certainly one will be manipulated. A physician on the other hand would consider alternative diagnoses and other methods of treatment as well as manipulation.

Orthopaedic surgeons will sometimes perform manipulations under anaesthetic. Sometimes they do this with a very light degree of anaesthesia such that the person is half awake. This is particularly helpful when it is uncertain how much back pain is due to damage in the spine and how much to an anxiety state. In the latter the relaxation provided will usually allow much greater freedom of movement. When the patient is completely asleep it is possible to stretch the spine fully and break adhesions limiting the movements of various joints. Orthopaedic surgeons use this technique carefully as sometimes it can stir up trouble rather than relieve pain. In the right person however, it can rapidly improve the movements of a stiff back. However, the majority of manipulations are performed with the patient fully awake so that he can describe the immediate results of the treatment. He will indicate whether there is relief of pain or the symptoms are aggravated. The techniques are constantly modified to provide the best results.

Many physiotherapists learn how to manipulate. In this

country, physiotherapists do not take patients directly but only by referral from a doctor. This ensures that a proper assessment is performed to make sure that nothing serious is being missed and that physiotherapy treatment is appropriate. There are great advantages in close co-operation between physiotherapists and doctors and the two professions work together each exploiting the skills of the other.

Although physiotherapists may learn any of the techniques of manipulation they usually practise the methods described by Geoffrey Maitland, a physiotherapist in Adelaide, Australia. The techniques are colloquially known as Maitland's mobilization and manipulation. The treatment entails repeated visits over several weeks with detailed assessment of the back during each session in order to localize the level responsible for the symptoms and to follow the patient's progress (Plate 5).

The treatments are directed at the particular level of the spine involved, although inevitably they also affect the adjacent levels, and the programme is modified according to progress. The most important component of treatment is mobilization, which consists of oscillatory movements applied manually to the vertebrae. These movements include rotation and backwards and forwards and side-to-side movements. They may be combined with manipulation techniques which are rapid movements of small amplitude going beyond the normal active ranges of motion. Sometimes traction is added. There may be exercises and occasionally local heat. Although Maitland described the general programme many physiotherapists will modify the treatment according to their own particular beliefs.

Of all the different forms of manipulation only that practised by physiotherapists has been tested by the scientific method. For such a study patients considered suitable for this treatment either receive manipulation or an innocuous type of therapy that superficially appears similar but in fact does not do anything. By comparing the progress of the two groups it is possible to assess the value of the trial treatment.

Back pain: the facts

I would like to describe two such studies with which I was personally concerned. The patients all had back pain. The first study was on back pain patients seeing their general practitioner and with symptoms that persisted long enough for a back X-ray to be requested. The second group had been referred by their general practitioner to hospital rheumatology or orthopaedic clinics for specialist opinions. These patients had more severe and persistent pain with greater disability and more severe X-ray changes. In each study the patients were randomly divided into two groups, one of which received mobilization and manipulation as described by Maitland and given by a physiotherapist who was specially experienced in these techniques. The rest were given a form of deep heat but with the machine turned down so low that no heat was produced. This was given by the same physiotherapist who tried to be as convincing as possible about this form of pseudo-treatment, although she realized it was ineffective. All treatments were given three times a week for as long as necessary up to four weeks. The progress of each patient was assessed by a doctor who did not know which type of treatment was being given. In this way any bias by the patient or by the doctor analysing the results was minimized.

In the general practitioner study the majority of patients, whether receiving manipulation or not, were much improved after the four-week treatment period. However those who received Maitland's mobilization and manipulation were slightly better than the rest. Two months later most patients were still improved but the differences between the two groups had largely disappeared. At final follow-up after a year the progress of the two groups was identical.

By contrast, in the hospital series, most patients were also improved after the four-week treatment period although they had not done as well as in the general practitioner study. This was expected as these patients had much more severe back problems. However, there was absolutely no difference in progress between those receiving manipulation or not.

Similarly two months later and at one year the progress of the two sub-groups was identical.

Information from the two studies was analysed very carefully. The conclusions were (a) that most episodes of back pain will get better; (b) that in those likely to improve, manipulation can hasten the process to a limited extent but it makes no difference in the long run; (c) that although some patients seemed to do well immediately after a mobilization and manipulation session other patients had similar improvement after a pseudo-treatment session. We even had one or two who came back asking for a further course of the pseudo-treatment when they developed another attack of back pain some time later. The patients in the hospital series had more severe problems and in these we failed to find any benefit from mobilization and manipulation.

So where does this leave mobilization and manipulation by physiotherapists? Most people will get better anyway. The treatment will accelerate improvement in a few. The personal attention and interest of the physiotherapist will play an enormous part in accelerating recovery. This will be dealt with in more detail with regard to the psychology of back pain in Chapter 11. The advice and instruction on the use and care of the back given during the treatment sessions is very helpful in avoiding future relapses. However the real value of the procedures themselves remains doubtful.

So the evidence in favour of mobilization and manipulation is pretty weak. It does suggest that it can have some temporary effect but it makes no difference in the long term. Nevertheless of all the trials published these studies provide the firmest evidence in favour of manipulation. Not even this limited evidence is available in favour of osteopathy or chiropractic. The use of a comparison group of patients who have not received the particular form of manipulation is remarkably chastening. If we had only treated patients with mobilization and manipulation and had not included a comparison group, we would have reported that about three-quarters of our patients got better and so decided that this was the treatment of choice. We now know that this is not so but simply that the natural powers of recovery of the back can be helped a tiny fraction by manipulation. It is up to the osteopaths and chiropractors to show that their forms of treatment are better. The challenge is there.

Should one seek manipulation?

So the position with respect to manipulation is very confused. Who should be manipulated? What techniques should be used? Should the manipulation be by physicians specializing in manipulative medicine, orthopaedic surgeons, physiotherapists, osteopaths, or chiropractors? Does it do any good? The evidence on these points has been presented and it is clear that the answers to these questions are not easy.

In the first place, one must be certain that the back pain is caused by a mechanical problem and not by some other disease that may be missed. Manipulation under such circumstances can be an absolute disaster. Bones may break, ligaments tear, and nerves be severely damaged, producing paralysis. A careful medical assessment is an essential preliminary and should be performed by a doctor who has the training to recognize these other causes of back pain. The diagnosis should be reviewed from time to time because a condition may not be obvious at its onset but becomes clear as time passes. Again medical assessments are essential. In the straightforward case, the careful examination and laboratory tests may seem a waste of time. Their importance lies in identifying the unusual problem and avoiding giving the wrong treatment.

Most attacks of back pain will get better with the more conservative forms of treatment already described. Manipulation may be the right answer for those who fail to improve but in my view the decision should be made by people with a medical training. After all, if one goes to an osteopath or chiropractor, one is seeking manipulation — one has already made the decision that one wants manipulation. Apart from the most exceptional circumstances that is what is given. Surely the patient should seek the best treatment, of which manipulation is only one of the options available? A balanced view of all the forms of treatment available is required.

Does manipulation do any good?

The lack of information about this has already been expressed. We hear many anecdotal stories of immediate recovery after manipulation but also of many others who failed to improve and some who are made worse. The evidence available suggests that most attacks of back pain will get better anyway; manipulation can hasten this in a few but it makes no difference in the long run and it does not prevent future attacks of back pain. The many different forms of manipulation and types of manipulators create further problems. We simply do not know if any one form of treatment is any better or worse than others. Proper, scientifically controlled trials are urgently required to answer these questions.

So in my view a medical assessment is essential and the decision about this form of treatment should only be made by someone with all the skills required. We simply do not know which type of manipulation is best but it may be worth trying for some cases. The results of further work trying out these various forms of treatment are eagerly awaited.

Lumbar corsets and spinal supports

If it hurts to move the back then splinting it in some form of support should relieve the symptoms. This simple concept led to the use of plaster-of-Paris spinal jackets and various types of spinal brace and lumbar corsets for back pain.

The plaster-of-Paris jacket is the most effective but is physically uncomfortable and can be worn only for a limited period. It is usually used for people with severe pain who must be able to get about and cannot receive complete bedrest as described earlier. Wet plaster-of-Paris bandages are wrapped over a body stocking. They set within a few minutes to form a solid shell that prevents the back moving. There are obvious difficulties with hygiene and washing so that this type of jacket can only be worn for a relatively short period of time.

On the other hand, spinal corsets are very widely used (see Plate 6). In Great Britain in one year about 400 000 lumbar corsets were prescribed under the National Health Service. This does not take into account corsets obtained privately or by patients themselves. This means that the total must be a staggering half million or so. Interestingly corsets are prescribed twice as frequently in England than in Scotland. We do not know why this is — perhaps the Scots are hardier.

There are many different manufacturers of lumbar corsets. They all make them to a common basic pattern but with considerable variation in style, form, materials, and fastenings. They all contain a strong strengthening pad which stretches from the sacrum to the mid-back and which is encased within a firm body belt which is tied around the abdomen. Most corsets use steel strips to provide the actual support and these are moulded to the shape of the patient's back. A recent design uses a heat-mouldable plastic pad. This is heated to 70 °C and moulded to the patient's back. On cooling it retains this shape but sets extremely firm. The pad is inserted in a special pocket in the back of the corset. The material of the corset is made of various types of cloth or even canvas. It must be strong to allow the corset to be drawn tight. For people who tend to get too hot, or for use in hot climates, there is a version available with multiple perforations which allow air to circulate. The corset is drawn tight with laces, straps, or special Velcro fastenings.

Wearing a corset will relieve pain in the back but does nothing for the underlying problem, so it is only a form of palliation. Indeed, it can do harm, as the muscles can become weak with lack of use and sometimes prolonged wearing of a corset can lead to the 'stuck back' described earlier. Corsets should be worn only for short periods, not indefinitely. When someone is starting to get going after a severe episode of back pain, and perhaps after being confined to bed, then the lumbar corset may help him to start moving around without upsetting his back. A corset may also be worn for a few days to help the patient over a mild attack of pain. However, many patients wear their corsets for months or years. Although they believe it helps them it can also prolong the whole back problem.

There are two theories as to how corsets work. The first is simply that they limit the back movement. The second is that the tightness of the corset raises the pressure with the abdomen so allowing it to transmit some of the body load and therefore decreasing that on the spine as described in Chapter 1. Although a certain amount of back movement can still be performed despite wearing the corset, it does appear that the limitation of the back movements is important and probably both mechanisms have a role to play in providing relief.

6

Pain and its control

Introduction

Although we all know what pain is, it is almost impossible to describe it adequately in words. It is an unpleasant type of sensation produced by injury or disease. We feel pain in our minds although we locate it in the affected part of the body. Without the conscious mind, pain would not exist, only a variety of electrical and chemical impulses.

Although pain is unpleasant it does serve an important purpose. It provides a warning that tissues are being damaged so that the subject can take appropriate action. If this ability to perceive pain is lost, injuries may occur without the subject being aware of it. Extreme cases of this are seen in certain neurological diseases in which loss of pain sensation in the fingers may allow them to be burned by cigarettes, or if feeling is lost in the feet poorly fitting shoes may rub and produce nasty ulcers.

One approach to the problem of back pain is not to worry too much about what is wrong with the back but simply to try to control the sensation of pain. In its simplest form, we use pain-relieving medicines like aspirin. However, modern advances in the understanding of the physiology of pain sensation are not only providing us with insight into how traditional forms of treatment may work but also leading to the development of new methods of pain control.

Pain-relieving medicines

Medicines that relieve pain are known as analgesics. They are often used for people with back pain and the particular ones prescribed will depend upon the severity and nature of the symptoms. In the patient with really severe back pain and sciatica, perhaps due to a burst intervertebral disc, very strong analgesics may be required. Sometimes even morphine or related drugs are used if they are the only drugs powerful enough to provide adequate relief of pain. There is a risk of addiction with medicines such as these. They have an obvious and important role for people dying from some very painful illness but doctors do not like using them for treating a non-fatal condition such as back pain. They are therefore used very sparingly, restricted to the most severe cases, withdrawn after a very short period of time, and replaced by simpler analgesics. However, recent research has shown that natural morphine-like substances (see p. 102) are formed within the brain and play an important role in controlling the actual experience of pain. More of this later.

Some analgesics are pain relievers alone but others also can reduce inflammation. These are known as non-steroidal anti-inflammatory analgesics. This means that they are not cortisone-like drugs and they can control inflammation as well as relieving pain. Although the anti-inflammatory effect is most obviously useful in inflammatory diseases like rheumatoid arthritis, there is an element of inflammation in many back problems so that these drugs are more valuable than pure pain relievers.

The most well known of the non-steroidal anti-inflammatory pain-relieving drugs is aspirin, which is technically known as acetyl salicylic acid. This drug was first extracted from the willow tree or salix — hence the name salicylates. Aspirin is a useful drug and is quite good at relieving pain. However, its effects last only a few hours and often it is necessary to take three tablets four times a day, or even more, to control the symptoms properly.

There is no medicine known that is without risk of possible side-effects. If one thinks about it, this is hardly surprising, because in order to be effective drugs must alter the ways in which cells and tissues in the body behave and such changes, if taken to excess, are likely to be harmful. Aspirin is no exception but fortunately, on the whole, it is a very safe drug. Many tons of aspirin are consumed per year and only a few people come to real harm. However aspirin can upset some people. The commonest problem is indigestion due to irritation of the stomach lining. Some patients may lose blood, either as a very slow process which may gradually produce anaemia or very occasionally as a sudden internal haemorrhage. An excessive intake of aspirin may cause ringing noises in the ears and even deafness, which improve once the dose is reduced.

In order to make the drug more acceptable aspirin is often presented in other forms. Perhaps the most popular is aspirin which can be dissolved in water. Sometimes the tablet has a special coating to prevent irritation of the stomach lining. It may be mixed or combined with other medicines in an effort to enhance its actions and to reduce some of the stomach upsets. Commonly I prescribe simple soluble aspirin, as many of the other preparations, particularly the extremely expensive forms sold under various brand names, have relatively little advantage over it.

If aspirin produces stomach upset, paracetamol is a useful alternative. It is not quite as effective a pain reliever as aspirin but carries less risk of an abdominal upset and for that reason is preferred by many people. Many of the preparations available contain mixtures of aspirin and paracetamol. There is one interesting compound in which the two are chemically combined and only separate once the drug is absorbed into the body, so providing dual benefit and avoiding some of the stomach problems of aspirin.

In an effort to improve on the performance of these pain-relieving compounds pharmaceutical companies have developed a whole new range of drugs, which are very similar to each other. Many of these compounds are related in their structure to propionic acid, and include ibuprofen (Brufen), naproxen (Naprosyn), ketoprofen (Orudis), diclofenac (Voltarol), fenclofenac (Flenac), azapropazone (Rheumox), and many others. The stimulus for their development was the need to control inflammation in diseases such as rheumatoid arthritis. However, they are also useful for back troubles and are often prescribed. They are as good or even slightly better than aspirin in relieving pain but have advantages in that they produce fewer stomach upsets, and fewer tablets have to be taken each day.

Indomethacin (Indocid) and phenylbutazone (Butazolidin) are better pain-relieving anti-inflammatory drugs than those mentioned so far. However they do carry a somewhat greater risk of unwanted effects. These include abdominal upsets of various sorts, and phenylbutazone rarely may affect the blood. Indomethacin can produce very unpleasant headaches and a feeling of muzziness. For these reasons these two drugs are usually reserved for the more severe back problems when other medicines do not have sufficient effect.

Pure pain-relieving drugs that have no anti-inflammatory properties are sometimes used. The more potent ones are available only on a doctor's prescription and include dihydro-codeine (DF 118) and dextroproproxyphene (Distalgesic, familiarly known as DG). Care must be taken with these drugs as too large a dose can be dangerous.

It is not possible to give a comprehensive account listing all the possible drugs as there is such a wide range available. However the majority fall within the broad groups or are related to those that have been described.

The way the tablets are taken depends upon the nature of the back problem. If the patient is continuously in pain then he should take them regularly throughout the day. If the pain is worse at any particular time of day then the medicine should be timed to be taken, say half or one hour before. Some people have a great deal of pain in bed at night. The first thing to do is to improve the bed but, if this is not ade-quate, then a larger dose of pain-relieving medicines last thing before going to sleep may prove the answer. Many of these tablets are effective only for three or four hours which means their benefits will have worn off by the early hours of the morning. There are now longer-acting tablets and also slow-release preparations available that lengthen the duration of action.

Another alternative which is aesthetically unappealing but which can be remarkably effective is to take the medicine in the form of a suppository. The chemicals are absorbed only very slowly from the back passage so that they work over a long period. Suppositories have another advantage in that they reduce the risk of abdominal upsets. For the person who suffers from severe indigestion, suppositories may be the answer. If I think a suppository may help I usually ask the patient to give them a try for a few days and then to discard them if they find the technique unacceptable or ineffective. The vast majority are so pleased with the results that they are happy to continue.

The perception of pain

For countless centuries opium has been used as a drug of addiction. Opium is derived from a certain species of poppy. The poppies grown in this country do not produce the drug but the seed pods of a special variety known as *Papaver somniferum*, which grows in warmer climates, produce quite large amounts. The drug may be taken by mouth but quite commonly it is smoked. A pipe is passed from person to person in communal sessions. The drug has a calming and relaxing effect and removes many anxieties. Frequent use may lead to a dependence on the drug, a requirement for greater quantities, and eventually to addiction. Use of opium and drugs derived from it is outlawed in most countries of the world. Although the basic constituents are remarkably easy to produce and extremely cheap, on the black market the drug costs many hundred or even thousand times its true value.

The active substance in opium that provides its effects is morphine. By simple chemical manipulation an even more potent substance, di-methyl morphine or heroin may be made. These compounds would be of purely legal interest but for the fact that they are the most potent pain-relieving substances known. They are effective in relieving severe pain when commonplace drugs such as aspirin have failed. Morphine and related chemicals are used for people suffering from severe pain, and particularly if they have a fatal illness. The most common of these is widespread cancer. Often they are used after operations when the need is to relieve pain for only a short period. The use of these drugs is always balanced against the potential risks of producing addiction and if this seems at all likely then extreme care is required.

All this may seem of academic interest with regard to back pain, as the majority of sufferers do not have sufficiently severe symptoms to merit the use of such drugs. However, in recent years there have been fascinating discoveries of how the brain perceives the sensation of pain and we have now come to realize that morphine-like substances are formed naturally within the brain and control our normal experience of pain.

Until very recently, ideas of pain perception had changed little over countless centuries. The common idea was that a stimulus felt peripherally such as a burn or a cut would stimulate special receptors in the skin which would convey a message along the nerves right up to the brain, thus producing the sensation of pain. The system was seen as a bit like a telephone line with a single wire that conveyed this special message – pain. Though this explanation accorded with the anatomical descriptions of the pathways of the nerves, nevertheless it failed to explain all the problems. Some of us may find a certain injury painful whereas others may tolerate it without significant discomfort. In other words we may have a low or high threshold to painful stimuli. Perhaps this just reflects the sort of people that we are. Some of us feel pain more readily than others. However, there is more to it than this as on some occasions we may find a particular stimulus excruciatingly painful yet on other occasions we may barely notice it. Perhaps the most graphic examples of this are soldiers in the heat of a battle or boxers during a fight, who may receive severe injuries and yet not notice them and continue fighting. It is only some time after the fight that they realize their injuries and feel pain.

David Livingstone, the nineteenth-century explorer in Africa, provided a remarkably vivid account of an incident very suggestive of a similar phenomenon. Livingstone was standing alone on a small grassy hill when he was suddenly attacked by a large male lion. He wrote:

I heard a shout. Staring and looking half round, I saw the lion just in the act of springing upon me. I was on a little height; he caught my shoulder as he sprang and we both came to the ground below together. Growling horribly close to my ear, he shook me as a terrier does a rat. The shock produced a stupor similar to that which seems to be felt by a mouse after the first shake of a cat. It caused a sort of dreaminess in which there was no sense of pain nor feeling of terror, though quite conscious of all that was happening. It was like what patients partially under the influence of chloroform describe, who see all the operation but feel not the knife. This singular condition was not the result of any mental process. The shake annihilated fear, and allowed no sense of horror in looking round at the beast. The peculiar state is probably produced in all animals killed by carnivora; and if so, is a merciful provision by our benevolent Creator for lessening the pain of death. (Livingstone (1872) *Adventures and discoveries in the interior of Africa*. Hubbard, Philadelphia.)

Livingstone is describing in himself and in animals an inappropriate tranquillity and lack of feeling of pain while being literally eaten alive. This has often been observed in animals and ascribed to 'a state of shock' without any real understanding of what has happened.

A simple telephone-line theory of pain-transmission cannot explain what is going on here. A certain stress should always produce the same unpleasant sensation and this would not be prevented by the circumstances in which the injury occurred.

Thus there seems to be some mechanism within the brain by which the sensation of pain can be suppressed in appropriate circumstances. This ability to suffer injury and not experience pain during periods of stress allows the subject to perform tasks or undertake procedures that otherwise he would be unable to do. The short-term advantage is that the soldier or boxer can fight on despite injury (although in the long run more harm than good may be achieved as pain usually provides a warning that should be heeded).

This phenomenon was regarded as little more than a curiosity until the late 1960s, when experiments were performed on animals in which parts of the brain were stimulated using minute electric currents, in the search for the various centres that control certain types of sensation. The particular one being sought was that responsible for pleasure. How fortunate we would be if by switching on this current we could stimulate such a centre in the brain and feel happy and contented! During the course of these experiments the scientists found that stimulating a certain part of the brain made the animal unresponsive to a painful stimulus although in other respects it remained normal. This discovery was applied to man and used for patients with severe pain uncontrollable by simpler means. The most common cause of this is extensive cancer. When electrodes were placed in the appropriate part of the brain and electrically stimulated there was a fading away of the pain. Nevertheless the patients remained fully awake and alert. Other sensations such as touch remained normal and the patients had full control over their bodily movements. These electrodes were tried in various regions and it was found that the most effective site was in the midbrain around the so-called central canal. The site was identical in both animals and in man.

This technique has been so successful that in some centres it is in use as a clinical form of pain control. The electrodes are placed in the right spot by insertion through a needle under three-dimensional X-ray control. They are left there permanently with the leads led away under the surface of the skin. Repeated electrical stimulation may be required. In some people they may be effective in controlling the pain for years. Although they do nothing to affect the cancer, this technique may well make the final period of the patient's life comfortable.

At the same time as this work was being developed further research was undertaken on morphine and drugs related to it.

In particular it was found that by a relatively trivial modification of the morphine molecule, a compound called nalorphine could be developed that blocked the effect of morphine
itself. That meant that if it was given prior to morphine then
the pain-relieving and other effects of morphine would disappear. This is not just a scientific curiosity but indicates that
within the brain there is a very specific receptor to which
morphine and allied drugs will attach to produce their effects.
When a compound that is similar but not quite the same is
given first, it can attach itself without producing morphine-
like effects and prevent the morphine molecule from subsequently combining with the same receptor.

The search was on to find where morphine and its blocking
agent worked. It is possible to attach markers to molecules so
that we can identify what happens to them inside the body.
In the case of morphine this is a radioactive hydrogen atom
which replaces one of the hydrogen atoms that is normally
present in the molecule. By giving the labelled drug to an
animal it is then possible to seek out where the label ends up.
Radio-labelled morphine was found in precisely the same area
in the midbrain, around the central canal, where electrical
stimulation gave pain relief.

The precise coincidence of these two areas was too much
to accept as a chance finding. It suggested that the two were
inherently related to each other. The possibility was raised
that morphine works by binding to particular receptor sites
in that region of the brain. Moreover the electrical stimulation
releases a morphine-like substance within that particular area
and that is why this technique is able to produce profound
control of painful sensation. This implies that the brain itself
is able to make a morphine-like substance. The next step was
to try to find the actual material and in 1975 workers in
Scotland for the first time identified morphine-like material
in the brain and called it enkephalin. We now know that
there is not a single morphine-like substance but a number of
substances known as endorphins and that they are principally
formed in this particular area of the brain.

Pain and its control

It has become apparent that there is a very complex system for controlling the sensation of pain. Not only will peripheral damage give rise to impulses that travel up the nerves to the brain to produce this sensation but also the brain itself has a mechanism for modulating the actual sensation experienced. Even this system has its complications and today our understanding of the subject is still rapidly expanding. We now know that there are fibres in the spinal cord that will preferentially stimulate this pain-controlling centre and prevent the sensation of pain. There are also fibres that descend from the pain-suppression centre down the spinal cord and will control the transmission of impulses between the nerves and the spinal cord itself. There are receptors in the spinal cord that respond to endorphins of the same sort as in the brain.

We now understand much more about how morphine can produce such profound control of pain. It is not simply a compound derived from the poppy that happens to be a pain reliever. It is a substance that mimics a naturally occurring material within the nervous system itself and that is why it has such profound effects. This suggests that the variability of pain actually experienced may be due to altered release of endorphins which occurs irrespective of the severity of the actual injury itself. If we can find ways of triggering the release of the naturally occurring endorphins then we may have a mechanism of pain relief that mimics that naturally occurring in the body.

Some of the pain-relieving methods that at first sight do not seem to have a proper scientific basis could well work by this mechanism. To take a simple example, if a child injures his leg his mother may be able to 'rub it better'. What happens when she does this? It seems very unlikely that the rubbing can do anything for the injury itself. We now believe that the rubbing stimulates certain nerves that run to the spinal cord and from there up to the pain-controlling centre in the midbrain and release the morphine-like substance, so providing relief of the symptoms.

We now know that stimulation of the skin produces

impulses that carry messages in nerves in both thin and thick fibres. Only the thin fibres convey the pain message but impulses in the larger fibres can block the perception of the painful element of the sensation. This is known as the gate control theory of pain. There is a 'gate' in the brain which is either open to allow pain to be felt or closed by stimulation of these large nerve fibres so that the pain disappears. It is a bit like a signal from a jamming station blocking reception of a radio broadcast. Many forms of treatment may work by closing the gate. These include massage, friction, mustard baths, ointments that produce some irritation of the skin, transcutaneous nerve stimulation (see p. 109), and even acupuncture. Clearly a fundamental readjustment of our ideas of pain control is well underway.

The study of the pain-controlling centre has also influenced our understanding of the placebo response. A placebo is a drug or technique which mimics a standard procedure under trial but in effect does nothing. We know that many back pain sufferers will seemingly respond well to a placebo, although the benefits generally are transitory. In the past the response to a placebo has usually been taken as an indication of the lack of any serious underlying problem. It was assumed that if someone got better when in truth nothing had been done then the problem was all in the mind and nothing serious was wrong in the first place. Evidence is emerging that this is a gross oversimplification. A series of patients who had undergone surgery were given a placebo which basically was a medicine totally lacking in effect, and half of them also received the morphine-blocking substance nalorphine. The pain was considerably worse in the group receiving nalorphine than in those receiving placebo alone. This suggests that the placebo is not doing nothing but can relieve pain by causing the release of morphine-like endorphins in the brain. The placebo benefit was blocked by the nalorphine in those receiving this drug.

Can endorphins be given by mouth and will they relieve pain and be useful for backache? The drug companies are just commencing research programmes along these lines. Already synthetic endorphins are available and have been found capable of producing profound pain relief when injected around the spinal cord. The latest compounds look promising for oral administration but it is still very early days to know how effective they will be, whether they will be useful for back pain and what complications may arise.

So there the matter rests at the present time. We are now beginning to appreciate how the central nervous system itself is able to alter the subjective experience of the sensation of pain by controlled release of endorphins. This knowledge is leading to new ideas on pain control.

Acupuncture

Acupuncture has been the subject of controversy for many years. It was used by the Chinese as a method of pain relief and to control a wide variety of different diseases. Until very recently acupuncture was totally disregarded by Western Medicine as unscientific and valueless. However, more enquiring approaches have provided support for a pain-relieving action under certain circumstances.

Techniques of acupuncture have been used since pre-history and there are records of acupuncture on bone etchings from about 1600 B.C. The first detailed description in Ancient Chinese literature was in *The Yellow Emperor's Book of Internal Medicine* written between 400 and 200 B.C. This book is written as a dialogue between the Yellow Emperor and a physician but probably represents a collection of teachings from around that time. The Yellow Emperor himself is believed to have lived at around 250 B.C. The Ancient Chinese believed in the principle of Tao — the Way — which was responsible for creating order out of chaos and the harmonious coexistence of good and evil. They believed in a vital essence or life force which they called Ch'i. This force might be called life energy and flows through all living things and is essential to their well-being. Ch'i is a balanced mixture of two opposing forces known as Yin and Yang. Yin is the negative, feminine, and passive force, while Yang is positive, masculine, and active. Examples of Yin things are night, autumn or winter, cold and the moon, and Yang things are day, spring or summer, heat and the sun. However, Yin and Yang are not exclusive but co-exist and blend with each other in complex ways.

The Ch'i or life force was believed to flow around the body through ducts, the lines of which were known as Meridians. There were twelve principal Meridians divided into two groups. One group of Meridians is Yang and is connected to the hollow organs of the body concerned with nutrition and excretion such as the gall bladder, the intestine and the bladder. The other Meridians are Yin and are related to the solid organs concerned with circulation of the blood such as the heart, lungs, liver, spleen, and kidney. The life force circulates through the Meridians in a definite order and at particular times of day and if the circulation is stopped or out of balance then sickness or death can result.

Detailed examination of the pulse at the wrist will tell whether there is any imbalance between the Meridians. The pulse in each hand is felt in three positions and palpated first with a very light superficial pressure and then with a much firmer grasp. This produces a total of twelve pulses and each will reflect problems in a different bodily organ. Analysis of the pulse is used to indicate what is wrong and to help in choosing the site for insertion of the acupuncture needles.

When it is known which Meridian is abnormal, the flow of Ch'i is corrected by inserting the needle in the acupuncture point on the Meridian. Complex charts were drawn by the ancient Chinese physicians showing not only these principal Meridians but other less important lines and showing the appropriate acupuncture sites for various disorders (Plate 7).

The traditional acupuncture needle was made of gold or silver and was of varying lengths, thicknesses, and shapes of point. Different schools of acupuncture inserted them at various depths. They could be inserted quickly or slowly, removed immediately or left in place, withdrawn, and re-inserted, and rotated clockwise or anti-clockwise, quickly or slowly. Some even put a blob of inflammable material known as moxa on the end of the needle. When lit it burned slowly and heated the needle and the skin. Some patients were treated only once and others daily. It is not clear whether these variations made any difference. Acupuncture was used for a wide variety of different disorders including not only back pain but also heart troubles, migraine, toothache, painful periods, and many other problems.

An interesting variant developed by French and Chinese acupuncturists was known as auriculo-therapy or ear acupuncture. According to the proponents of this system, the whole body is represented upside-down on the surface of the ear. By palpating the ear and today, by using electrical tests, they believe they can diagnose which part of the body is abnormal. This area is treated by acupuncture.

Acupuncture is still frequently used for back pain although its real value remains in doubt. Although many patients will claim relief of pain after this treatment the evidence obtained by comparing patients treated properly and by sham or incorrect acupuncture techniques has shown that there is little if any advantage for those treated in the official acupuncturist's manner. It may be that the precise site of insertion of the acupuncture needles does not matter too much, so that correctly or incorrectly performed acupuncture may still provide the same benefit. Perhaps it is the needling that counts irrespective of the ancient Chinese theories. If the technique works, and it does seem to help in some people, it provides only temporary pain relief but will not alter the underlying fault and is not of long-term value. In those who benefit, the relief from pain may last anything from a few hours to several weeks.

Today acupuncturists often use stainless steel needles. The needles must be properly sterilized to avoid transmitting disease. Acupuncturists often stick to the traditional acupuncture sites although many do this out of custom rather than belief. Sometimes they measure the electrical resistance of the skin, as alterations are thought to indicate where the needles are best inserted. Others may use the traditional sites indicated by pulse diagnosis. An examination may be made for tender trigger spots and the needles inserted there (Plate 8). Stimulation is performed by either rotating the needle or sometimes by passing a small electric current. Patients may report a sensation called 'take' derived from the Chinese word 'Te-Ch'i' which is a numb sensation developing around the acupuncture site. When a 'take' occurs the results are likely to be good.

There are various theories about how acupuncture can relieve pain. One idea is that it is simply a form of hypnotic suggestion and that the procedure itself is relatively unimportant. It is more likely that the needling stimulates the large nerve fibres that travel up to the brain and will block the transmission of pain impulses conducted through small nerve fibres, so closing the 'gate' described earlier. When acupuncture was done in an area previously rendered devoid of sensation by infiltrating with local anaesthetic, the pain-relieving action of the acupuncture itself was lost. Acupuncture could cause the release of endorphins in the midbrain, so preventing perception of pain. It is a fascinating discovery that the relief of pain by acupuncture is abolished by the morphine-blocking drug nalorphine. If endorphins are released in the midbrain by acupuncture it is fortunate that they are non-addictive as otherwise we might well find vast numbers of people totally committed to acupuncture stimulation. The successful treatment by acupuncture of withdrawal symptoms in some cases of heroin and morphine addition may well work in this way.

So the current evidence is that acupuncture can provide relief of pain. It is probably the needling that counts and the precise site is relatively unimportant. However, the method will only give temporary relief of symptoms and not for everybody. Although of some help it is not satisfactory in the long-term management of the back pain problem.

Pain and its control

Transcutaneous nerve stimulation

Pain relief from acupuncture arises by stimulation of the skin. Because of the physical difficulty in inserting needles, an electrical method known as transcutaneous nerve stimulation or TNS has been developed. Tiny pulses of electricity are applied to the skin with the aim of stimulating the large nerve fibres and closing the 'gate' in the brain, so preventing the passage of pain impulses and relieving the sensation of pain.

The apparatus consists of a small portable case containing a battery and controls with leads connected to electrodes which are attached to the body. The skin is cleaned thoroughly and dried. The electrode pads are covered with a special electrically conducting jelly and taped to the skin. Controls on the stimulator will adjust the severity of each impulse, the frequency with which they occur, and the length of time that each impulse lasts. The pulses are felt as pricking sensations and the controls adjusted to provide the most comfortable level. The site of the pain will usually determine where the electrodes should be fixed. Often it is a matter of trial and error to determine where they are most effective. The stimulator is worn on a belt or carried in a pocket and the patient can carry on with normal activities and simply switch on the apparatus whenever the need arises (Plate 9). The actual current flowing is minute and cannot produce burns or any local damage. However, there is a risk in people with heart pacemakers as the electrical pulses may interfere with their function. In general they are inadvisable for such patients. In people with other types of heart disease they can affect the heart rhythm and they should be used only after careful evaluation.

Some patients can obtain remarkable relief of pain by TNS and after each burst of impulses this may last anything from a few minutes up to several days. It is often difficult to know who will benefit and in a comparison between TNS and a sham device for sufferers from intractable low back pain there was no real advantage for the stimulator. However some people are convinced that they are helped and for them this is good enough.

This is still a rapidly advancing field with improvements in techniques constantly appearing. I am sure that we can look forward to considerable developments in this type of approach to pain control.

7

Injections and operations

This chapter is about highly specialized forms of treatment for back pain. They require very careful assessment of the back problem by skilled physicians and surgeons who are practised in the various techniques. In general, injections and operations are reserved for more severe back problems when simpler forms of treatment have not worked.

Injections for low back pain

Injections are used in several different ways for low back pain sufferers. They may be made into trigger points, into the epidural space, or directly into the intervertebral disc.

Trigger points and fibrositic nodules

Some patients have well-defined very tender areas in the back. They are best identified by carefully feeling the back with the patient lying on his stomach. Often a small firm nodule can be felt in the muscle. These nodules can be exquisitely tender and pressing on them makes the back pain very much worse. When the right area is found, the patient will make it known in no uncertain fashion.

These tender areas are known as trigger points, as pressure triggers the symptoms; they are sometimes called fibrositic nodules. Nobody knows what these nodules are and what actually happens at trigger points. Years ago it was thought that they were tiny pieces of fat that had burst through the sleeve of tissue around the muscle. Another idea was that the muscle had gone into spasm at that point because of damage to a nerve in the spinal column. Whatever the reason it is often worth trying an injection into a tender trigger point.

111

As the needle must hit the exact spot that is tender, the injection process itself can be very painful, but the patient is (or should be) comforted by the information that if the injection hurts and particularly if it stirs up the actual complaint itself it is more likely to be helpful in the long run. If the injection is painless, the trigger point probably has been missed and a good result is unlikely.

The injection usually consists of a small quantity of a cortisone-like drug mixed with local anaesthetic. Cortisone-like drugs given in this way do not cause the unpleasant side-effects that may happen if steroids are taken regularly, especially in a large dose. The local anaesthetic will 'deaden' or 'freeze' the tissues so that within two or three minutes the pain of the injection and of the complaint itself will disappear. However, the effect of the anaesthetic wears off within three or four hours and the pain may return. The real improvement hopefully will start within two or three days and the back pain can clear up completely in a week or so. Sometimes it only partially gets better and it is worth trying a second shot.

As we do not know what a trigger point is, it is hardly surprising that we are equally ignorant about how the injections work. It could be the anaesthetic, the cortisone, or indeed the needling itself acting as a type of acupuncture. Nevertheless some patients are very pleased with the results and as the method is so simple it is often worth trying.

Epidural injection

The technique of epidural injection is much more complex and used only for intractable problems when the back pain has failed to get better with other types of treatment already mentioned.

Within the spinal column and lining the vertebral canal is a tough layer of fibre-like tissue known as the dura. The spinal cord and nerve roots run down the canal inside the dura before they pass out between the vertebral arches. The epidural space lies outside the dura between it and the inner margins of the vertebral canal. In this form of treatment an injection is given directly into the epidural space.

Only doctors practised in the method use this technique. The epidural space is entered by a long needle inserted directly from behind, or passed upwards from just below the coccyx or tail bone. The injected material consists of a mixture of anaesthetic and a cortisone-like drug. Afterwards the patient will have to rest for at least an hour or two.

When it works, pain relief following this technique is immediate. In some people, however, it only lasts a few hours or days and then the pain comes back. If this happens, it may be worth trying a second epidural injection as this can have a longer-lasting effect.

The value of epidural injections was shown in a careful study performed in Guy's Hospital of 100 patients, half of whom received an epidural injection and the other half a sham injection. Those given the proper injection obtained greater relief of pain and more often returned to work. The Guy's doctors showed that this method can be useful for back pain, particularly if there is also sciatica.

Quite how the technique works is unknown. One suggestion is that the actual volume and pressure of the injected fluid breaks the small adhesions around the nerve roots, so freeing them. Another possibility is that with damage in the back there is some inflammation and swelling. The swollen tissues rub during back movements so causing more inflammation and swelling and the damage never has a chance to heal. Cortisone is so effective in controlling inflammation that the swelling clears, the rubbing stops, and the back pain clears up. Whichever, if either, of these theories is correct, this method of treatment does hold some promise and is currently undergoing further tests.

Dissolving damaged discs

Enzymes are biological catalysts, chemicals derived from animal or vegetable material which are capable of speeding up various chemical reactions which occur in the body. We use certain types of enzymes in washing powders as they hasten the dissolving of biological tissues and will rapidly remove stains from clothes.

One enzyme, chymopapain, which is obtained from the papaya or pawpaw fruit, is able to dissolve the nucleus of the intervertebral disc. An interesting experiment is to drop some disc material into a solution of chymopapain and watch it disappear over a few hours. On the basis of observations like this, chymopapain was injected into discs in an effort to dissolve them medically rather than remove them at a surgical operation. The technique is called 'chemo-nucleolysis', which means chemical lysis or dissolving of the nucleus. Because chymopapain is such a powerful enzyme, it is essential to be sure the injection is in exactly the right place as otherwise the wrong tissues might be dissolved. The procedure is performed under direct X-ray control with a small amount of X-ray contrast dye injected into the nucleus first to confirm the position of the needle tip in the nucleus before performing the special injection.

The preliminary results look very promising and if they hold up in long-term studies it is likely that chemo-nucleolysis will become more widely used. Most of us would prefer to be treated by injection than by an operation. However, it is still early days: the technique requires a very high degree of skill and the method is only available in a few very specialized centres.

One problem that has emerged is that some people are sensitive or allergic to chymopapain. Sensitization arises following some previous exposure to the chemical. Several centuries ago, the Polynesians at the time of feasts and festivals would wrap cuts of meat in papaya leaves to make them tender and succulent. Papain is an important component of meat tenderizers which are widely used today, particularly in the United States. It helps 'to ameliorate the hardships of an affluent but toothless society'. The reason is that the enzymes will dissolve the tough fibres in the meat so softening

114

it in the same way as chymopapain dissolves discs. Those who eat tenderized meat can become allergic to the chymopapain and then develop reactions following the injection. Skin rashes are the commonest problem. Fortunately meat tenderizers are used very little in Britain.

Facet joint nerve blocks

As pain can be produced by damage to the tiny facet joints between the vertebrae, the idea arose of blocking the nerves coming from these joints so that pain would no longer be felt. The original idea was developed in Australia and the technique was performed by trying to cut the nerves with a scalpel inserted through a tiny skin incision. The operation was performed without actually seeing the nerves and it is very doubtful whether all the nerves from the facet joints were cut. More recently injections of phenol, which kills the nerves, have been used instead of a surgical incision. Another idea is to insert a needle and heat it with radio-frequency waves to block the nerves.

The results of facet joint blocks have been very mixed. The actual techniques are constantly being improved but it is too soon to know whether the method will be of real value.

Surgery for low back pain

Although back pain is so common and patients are often seen by orthopaedic surgeons, the amount of actual back surgery performed is relatively small. It is the vast size of the back problem rather than the need for operations by individuals that leads to the enormous amount of surgery performed in our hospitals. Although many patients worry about operations for back pain the chances of one being necessary are very low.

To put things in perspective, most attacks of back pain are transient and get better without need of medical help. For every 100 000 bouts of back pain, it has been calculated that only 10 000 people consult their doctor. Most of these attacks will get better and the general practitioner will only refer about one in five or 2000 of these people to hospital rheumatology or orthopaedic clincs for a specialist opinion. Long waiting-lists unfortunately are not uncommon in British hospitals but an interesting benefit from this is that many back sufferers will recover while waiting to see the specialist. One estimate is that about two-thirds will get better in this way so leaving about 700 who are actually seen in the clinic. About one in ten or 70 of these would require admission to hospital. Most will recover with rest, physiotherapy, and medical treatment or are unsuitable for surgery and only one in ten of these or seven would need an operation. So we are left with a figure of about seven operations for every 100 000 attacks of back pain. This should be very comforting for those who fear that surgery will be required following their attack of back pain.

In the nineteenth century operations on the spine were usually for the correction of deformities. Only relatively recently has surgery for back pain become common. It was the discovery by Mixter and Barr in 1934 that discs can burst and damage nerve roots so producing back pain and sciatica that led to the development of surgical treatment. There was enormous enthusiasm for operations in the early years, in the belief that removal of the damaged disc would cure the problem. More recently this enthusiasm has become tempered by experience and operations are undertaken today only when there are very definite indications. The wrong operation can do more harm than good, so very careful assessment is necessary before taking this step.

First of all the precise cause of the pain must be known. It is no good just opening up the back on spec. and perhaps dealing with one disc, if that is not the cause of the trouble. Surgery is a very precise science and the precision arises because the operation will only affect the exact site at which it is performed. The difficulties in determining the source of back symptoms in many patients have already been discussed.

PLATE 6. A lumbo-sacral corset (by courtesy of Messrs Spencer (Banbury) Ltd).

足太陰脾經之圖

凡二十穴
左右共四十穴

上行俠咽

周榮
胷鄉
天谿
食竇
腹哀
大橫
腹結
府舍

大包

箕門
血海

陰陵泉
地機
漏谷
三陰交
商丘
太白
太都

公孫
隱白

圖五十八——仿明版古圖(四)

PLATE 7. Ancient Chinese acupuncture points (by courtesy of Dr. Felix Mann).

Injections and operations

If it is not possible to identify the precise nature of the problem, an operation should be avoided. The spine is so complex that the exact approach adopted by the surgeon is dictated by the actual procedure to be performed. With a burst disc, the exact site of the back pain and sciatica and the findings on physical examination indicate which disc is at the root of the trouble. The clinical diagnosis is usually backed up by specialized X-ray studies, including myelography. This information tells the surgeon whether an operation is likely to help and if he decides to proceed, where to make his incision and how to get at the offending part.

The pain and amount of disability must be severe enough to merit operation. In general, back problems for which surgery is recommended are not life-threatening although if the nerves to the bladder and bowel are damaged an operation may be required as an emergency. The indications for operation are not absolute but depend on the degree of suffering and interference with normal life. If the pain is so severe as to disturb sleep, is not controlled by adequate pain-relieving tablets, and leads to continued loss of work, then surgery may be advisable.

However, the operation is not performed as a first line of treatment. An adequate period of simple conservative treatment should be tried first. This may include complete bed-rest, physiotherapy, pain-relieving tablets, and other measures and only if the symptoms persist after an adequate trial should one go on to think about operations. How long is an adequate trial of bed-rest? Again there are no hard and fast rules, but if the pain is no better after three or four weeks of complete rest on a properly supported bed then it may be time to consider further measures.

Not everybody is suitable for operation. As surgery is not being undertaken as a life-saving measure, patients with severe heart or chest disease may be unsuitable subjects for a major anaesthetic. Personality problems also come into it. In people who suffer from depression, anxiety, or other psychiatric diseases it may be impossible to separate the back pain resulting

117

from the actual damage in the spine from symptoms exacerbated by psychological factors. In such people the results of operations can be poor and indeed many are made worse. On the other hand in someone with severe, unremitting back pain, depression and anxiety may simply be caused by the persistent nature of the problem and surgery may be the only hope. Very careful assessment is essential before going ahead with surgery under these circumstances.

Finally, the patient must want to have the operation. It is inadvisable to press reluctant patients into having an operation. Even with a successful operation there are often some trivial remaining problems and the reluctant patient may well not be satisfied. The wise surgeon will put the pros and cons to patients whom he thinks he can help but will only operate if the patient is keen to go ahead.

Almost all operations are performed using a general anaesthetic. The actual operation depends upon the individual problem. For a burst disc the vertebral canal is opened up and the damaged disc inspected. It is usually possible to see the burst as a knob of fibrous tissue pressing on the nerve root. The surgeon will remove not only the burst but also the whole disc itself. If only the burst is removed there is immediate relief of the pressure on the nerve root but a risk of a further recurrence as more material can be squeezed out from the damaged disc. At the same time the surgeon will make a decision about whether to fix the two vertebrae together. This is known as spinal fusion. If there is any tendency for a vertebra to slip forwards or backwards then he is likely to perform a spinal fusion. He will also look critically at the size and shape of the spinal canal. The problems of spinal stenosis and the ways of detecting it have been described in Chapter 4. Many patients with back pain and sciatica have smaller canals than normal, so placing them at special risk of damage to the nerve roots. Sometimes this narrowing is not obvious even at operation as the exit canals are located very much to the sides and are quite deeply hidden. The surgeon looks carefully for such narrowing and if it is found will remove enough bone to create more free space.

Injections and operations

Following a straightforward disc removal, most patients start standing and walking within a few days. Often they will wear a lumbar corset when they start to get going. They are instructed on the right ways to sit and lift and usually can return to light work within about four to six weeks. In general they are not fit for heavy manual jobs for at least three months and sometimes much longer.

Before undergoing an operation on their back most patients would like a guarantee of success. However, it is never possible to make absolute promises. There is no operation known with a 100 per cent guaranteed success rate. There is always a risk, however remote, of totally unexpected findings or difficulties apart from the actual problems of the operation itself. However, most patients for whom surgery is advised will be pleased with the results, although there will be a small percentage who are no better or are even worse following this treatment. There are risks attached to any surgical procedure. Even having dental treatment carries some hazard, admittedly minute, but there for all that. Complications of back surgery are very rare and probably occur in no more than 1 per cent of patients.

Most surgeons will put the facts to the patient before performing the operation so that the patient can make up his own mind about whether to have it done. In general, surgery is much better for the sciatic pain felt in the leg than for backache alone. As a rough guide, out of every ten patients, eight are completely relieved of leg pain but only about five or six of back pain. Although these figures do not seem quite as good as one might like, remember that many of these patients have the worst back problems and that other types of treatment have failed.

A decision about surgery requires careful thought by both the surgeon and the patient. However, if the indications are right, the chances of success are very high and the operation is well worth performing.

8

Prevention of back pain

Back pain affects most of the population sooner or later. There is more work lost in British factories from this cause than from virtually any other problem. On the basis of the old adage that prevention is better than cure, much effort has gone into identifying those most likely to suffer from back pain, the types of work likely to cause it, problems with posture at home and at work, and improving methods of undertaking various tasks. Such studies cover all aspects of human life and many of the problems interrelate in complicated ways. It is often difficult to identify the role of any single factor in production of back pain because of the complex associations with related problems. Nevertheless, progress has been made and we are able to provide a certain amount of advice and recommendations to minimize the back problem. There is still considerable scope for a more detailed understanding of how man interacts with his environment and develops back pain, for improving the advice that is available, and above all for seeing that this advice is actually put into practice.

Who gets back pain?

Sex seems to influence most aspects of our lives and the incidence of back pain is no exception. In industry, the problem is much more frequent in males than females. However, the explanation of this difference is not at all clear. It could be that the male spine is built differently from the female's and is damaged more easily. It seems more likely, however, that as men on the whole undertake heavier work than women they are more likely to damage their backs. Also, the same backache may allow someone to continue in a light job but not in heavy manual work.

Prevention of back pain

Measurements show that as a crude approximation women possess about 60–70 per cent of the strength of males. This is because women are generally not only smaller but also their bodies contain a somewhat higher proportion of fat and lower proportion of muscle. There is a greater incidence of back problems in those performing the heaviest work, who are mainly males, but in light to moderate work groups back problems are of similar frequency in both sexes. There is not much one can do about one's sex but these observations may well be a pointer in indicating the amount of physical activity the spine can stand.

Back problems affect all ages. The greatest incidence in industry occurs in those between 35 and 50 years old with a decline thereafter. This is quite surprising because it would seem likely that the gradual loss in strength occurring with ageing would put older workers at greater risk of back problems. There are several possible explanations. It could be that those with back troubles seek alternative lighter jobs as they get older so that only fit workers remain within heavy industry, or that the younger, less skilled, employees fail to recognize tasks beyond their physical abilities and so more readily injure themselves whereas the older workers treat such jobs with more respect.

Being overweight is an important risk factor. The excess must be carried by the trunk which is supported by the spine and so in the long run obesity can aggravate back problems. Overweight back sufferers should diet in order to get to their ideal weight. Losing weight is easier said than done. Like smoking, those who are afflicted recognize their problem but have difficulty in doing anything about it. I do not recommend crash diets which involve virtual starvation with a seemingly satisfying loss of weight occurring within the first few weeks. Experience shows that patients will only tolerate a crash diet for a relatively short period of time and sooner or later are unable to stand it any more. They succumb to a craving for food and after a hard struggle eventually regain all they have lost. I recommend a much more gradual

121

loss of weight by adopting a diet that can be lived with for life. By avoiding fats, cakes, sweets, chocolate, and sugar and refusing second helpings it should be possible gradually to slim down. It is important to avoid going hungry by eating regularly but not excessively.

The tall members of the population are also somewhat more likely to develop back pain than normal-sized people. This is probably because of the excess leverage they produce when bending forwards. There is nothing one can do about one's height; it simply remains a pointer in suggesting avoidance of excessive bending.

Pre-employment medical examinations

In an effort to minimize the back problem in industry, many applicants for jobs will face medical checks before they are finally accepted. Employers regard these as particularly important if the work involves heavy manual labour as they hope to avoid placing their workers in the wrong job by such means. They may well have a vested interest in trying to avoid paying workers lying in bed with a bad back and particularly in minimizing the risk of compensation claims in case the back pain is blamed on some incident occurring at work. The aim is to identify those most likely to develop back problems by the initial screening examination and either not take them on or give them some less arduous post.

Although such an approach may seem logical, unfortunately the results of pre-employment medical screening have been very disappointing. Other than the factors already mentioned there is little to find by physical examination to indicate likely back sufferers. The examination of the spine or indeed the whole body provides virtually no clues indicating who is at special risk. The only really helpful point is a previous history of back troubles. Someone who has had spinal problems before, and particularly if they have had several attacks of back pain, is likely to suffer further problems, especially if he has to perform heavy manual work. From the points of view of both the worker and the employer it is better that the back sufferer should undertake a job within his physical ability.

In some industries, the pre-employment examination included X-rays of the spine and used these to exclude potential back sufferers. Unfortunately the relation between X-ray changes and back pain is very poor and if all those who show some abnormality on the X-ray are refused there would be very few left to actually undertake the work. It is very doubtful whether X-rays can be used in this way and studies show little change in the size of the back pain problem with use of this screening technique. In a study in North America there was no difference in the X-rays of groups of workers without back troubles and those disabled by them. The issue is not settled, however. In a study in Minnesota, when the patients with gross X-ray changes were excluded from employment, there was a considerable fall in the incidence of back problems. However, this was at the cost of rejecting about 28 per cent of the applicants purely on these grounds and there must have been many who were refused work but never developed back pain.

In addition, spine X-rays require a high dose of radiation. Although this is necessary for some individuals with back problems, it is not acceptable as a mass screening technique, particularly as the results are of such doubtful value.

Back pain and industrial tasks

The alternative to trying to exclude the employee who might develop a bad back is to look at industry, identify the tasks that may produce back problems, and modify them accordingly. Although statistics are not altogether clear, there does seem a greater risk of low back pain for those involved in heavy industry and manual work. Interestingly, the incidence in nurses is equal to that of heavy industry, whereas policemen get off quite lightly. Although nursing might seem a relatively light occupation, it frequently involves considerable

Back pain: the facts

back strain in bending over beds and lifting ill patients. It is hard to believe that being a policeman confers special immunity to back problems; it is more likely that back sufferers leave the job quite rapidly and only those that are completely fit will remain.

Simply labelling industry as involving 'heavy' or 'light' work is extremely crude and superficial as there are so many different tasks within a single trade. In the coal mines the work varies from work at the coal face to transporting the coal, working the lifts, and even desk jobs in the office. Detailed analyses of individual occupations are more important.

For example, it has become clear that standing still in one spot continuously for hours at a time will lead to aches and pains, particularly in the back. There is a need to move about regularly and change position. On the other hand, sudden and unexpected movements are liable to damage the back and produce back pain. In a survey of over 3000 individuals, low back pain was much more frequent in those who often had to perform sudden maximal physical efforts than in those who rarely or never did so. Sudden twisting movements are particularly bad in this respect.

Because of the risks of heavy manual work, measurements have been made of the physical forces required for various jobs and comparing these with suggested maximum limits. The problem with legal limits on the maximum physical effort required in a job is that the way the task is performed can be as important as the load itself. Moreover, there is the implication that any effort within the prescribed limit is harmless. Repeated lifts of lesser weight may be equally damaging. Authorities who wish to play safe may set the limit so low that virtually no work can be done. The International Labour Office has suggested limits for weight-lifting in industry but there is no agreement about whether their figures have a valid basis. However, they did find that those involved in very heavy work had a three-fold increase in incidence of back, knee and shoulder problems, a five-fold increase in hip problems, and a ten-fold increase in elbow problems. In Britain the regulations about weight-lifting are somewhat indecisive, with the generalization that no one should be required to handle a load that is likely to cause injury. Certain industries have their own rules which often bear no relation to each other. However, there is general agreement that the maximum lift for adult males should be about 55 kg (120 lb). Nevertheless meat porters and dockers still carry sides of beef or bales of jute weighing over 100 kg (220 lb).

Simply measuring the weight to be lifted is a very crude way of determining the stress and risks for the back and takes little account of the circumstances and postures in which the effort is performed or the shape of the object being handled. For example, considerably greater stress is required for an object held at arms' length rather than close to the body. When objects are held above the head or shoulders, balance is more difficult and sudden movements may produce back pain. Lifting a compact load between the knees uses the powerful hip and thigh muscles and is far easier than raising it above waist height, which relies on the weaker shoulder and elbow muscles.

A new and interesting approach developed in Michigan involves comparison of the maximum force involved in the particular lift with the maximum that could be achieved by very strong workers in that identical posture. This provides a lift strength rating (LSR) which is defined as:

$$\text{LSR} = \frac{\text{maximum load lifted}}{\text{the predicted maximum lift capability}}.$$

When the job required an LSR of 0.2 or greater there was a considerable increase in the incidence of low back pain. The research provided charts showing the maximum strengths of large strong males in various positions and the physical forces required in particular tasks are compared with these. If the LSR is 0.2 or more then the job is altered to make it easier. This method provides a real advance in understanding the physical requirements of various types of manual labour and more widespread application should lead to the elimination of hazardous tasks and their replacement by more acceptable procedures.

However, the LSR test can only be applied to about 70 per cent of manual jobs. In the remaining 30 per cent the lifts do not readily fall into the patterns described because they are performed with one hand and unevenly and perhaps performed on moving objects. Further development of the method is going on.

Assessment of strength of employees

The more detailed tests of the physical requirements of various types of occupation has led to similar and more specific assessments of the strengths of employees performing particular tasks. Some of these tests are carried out in a standard fashion to measure the strength of the arms, legs, trunk, and so on. The subject is asked to pull or push on a measuring device which will record his physical ability. The alternative is to identify the most demanding component of the job by the lift strength rating test and observe his strength in that posture. This is with the aim of matching the employee to the particular job. An index called the employee strength rating (ESR) has been developed which is:

$$ESR = \frac{\text{weight of object lifted on job}}{\text{maximum employee strength in that job position}}.$$

Although it is still early days to know quite how useful ESR is, there is already preliminary evidence that jobs requiring a repeatedly high ESR are associated with back problems.

The focus has also shifted from studying individual workers to average workers on a particular job with a job strength rating (JSR) defined as:

$$JSR = \frac{\text{object weight lifted on job}}{\text{average maximum strength of workers in that job position}}.$$

Again early results suggest that the JSR may be helpful in indicating the risk of back problems.

Prevention of back pain

These and other similar tests are exciting approaches to the problem of back pain in industry. They point the way to determining jobs liable to cause back pain, developing better methods of performing the same task, and ensuring that individual employees are not asked to exceed their physical abilities.

Back pain is common in industry. Whether the work actually causes the pain or simply brings on the problems in a person with a weak back is often not very clear. Whichever is true, there are many workers who continue in unsuitable employment despite considerable back problems. The failure to change jobs or modify the working posture can be due to a number of factors. Amongst these are lack of good advice, inflexibility of working patterns, loyalty to comrades or employers, lack of alternative work, and financial constraints, as with coal-face workers recommended for other jobs in the colliery. A better understanding of the relationship between work practices and stress on the back should reduce the magnitude of the back problem in the future.

Standing

Prolonged standing at work and at home should be avoided. However, such advice often is not practical. Many jobs require the worker to be on his feet for much of the day. Back problems can be minimized by standing in the right way. Frequent changes of position are important and there must be room to move about and to stretch at frequent intervals. As far as possible the head should be kept up with the shoulders straight and the hollow in the low back preserved. Not only is this the most comfortable position but also it looks the most attractive. The slouch looks bad and also leads to overstretching of the ligaments of the spine and backache. High-heeled shoes tip the body forward and make one arch backwards to compensate. Although they may be fashionable, they should be avoided for prolonged use, particularly by back sufferers.

127

FIG. 15. Good (left) and poor standing postures

Prevention of back pain

Industry often requires its employees to undertake bench work. Standing and leaning over a bench with the back bent and insufficient room for the legs is a very effective method of producing backache. The height of the bench should allow the employee to work in the upright position. The right height to work is level with the elbow when the arm is hanging freely by the side of the body. The work surface should be about 8 cm below this. Below the bench there must be room for the feet, and the most comfortable position is with one foot in front of the other in order to assist balance.

FIG. 16. The right and wrong (left) ways to work at a bench

Lifting techniques

Practices to avoid are lifting objects above eye level, carrying heavy items at arms' length, which magnifies the effect of the weight, trying to lift badly shaped objects, and pulling and pushing at low levels. Careful thought and redesign of the job should reduce these problems.

Lifting is probably the most common single cause of

episodes of acute back pain. Apart from limiting the weight of the load, much research has gone into improving techniques of manual handling and lifting with training programmes now given in many industries.

The most common way of lifting is the free-style technique and is used by people who have received no instruction on how to lift. The knees are straight or slightly bent and the back is rounded. The spine is unsupported by the muscles and the ligaments are readily over stretched. The free-style lift of heavy objects is a potent cause of back problems. Until quite recently the straight back/bent knees method was regarded as the method of choice. The subject crouches down in front of the object with the back straight, grasps the object, and then lifts upright using the hip and thigh muscles. Despite initial enthusiasm considerable doubts have crept in about this method. The feet are close together producing a small base and an unstable starting position for the lift. The full flexion of the hips and knees needed to lift a heavy object from the floor causes the heels to rise so that only the front of the foot remains in contact with the floor. This makes the base smaller and the position even more unstable. The result is that the subject must concentrate on maintaining balance as well as the lift itself. It is this initial phase of raising the object off the floor which has led to the current doubts about the straight back/bent knees technique.

Following a great deal of thought and much practical experience, the kinetic lift method is believed to be the optimum way of lifting and is now taught in many industries. The principles of the technique involve keeping the back straight although not necessarily upright, the chin in, the right positions of the feet, a good grip on the object with the arms close to the body, and using the body weight to assist in moving the object. The method is taught in the factory by a demonstrator. He would usually start by explaining the back problems, the risks caused by faulty techniques, and the likely benefits from better handling methods. He obtains the respect of his audience by demonstrating how to move a heavy,

FIG. 17. Methods of lifting. A. Free style. B. The straight back/bent knees method. C. The recommended kinetic technique

awkward object such as a large oil drum and illustrates common faults such as poor grip, the free-style lift, and the effects of a poor foot position and follows this by teaching them the kinetic method applied to the various types of problem that the workers are likely to meet.

The first step is to size up the job and think whether or not the object is too heavy or bulky. If so, the task should be divided into two or more parts, another colleague should be asked to help, or a mechanical means of lifting should be used. The position of the feet is all-important. They should be spread about 50 cm (20 in) apart with one foot behind the object and the other by the side of the object and pointing in the direction in which it is to be moved. This has two benefits. The broad base is very stable and avoids balancing problems. By pointing the forward foot in the direction of travel, it will not be necessary to twist the spine when the object is lifted but simply to move the rear foot. The worker squats down with the hips, knees, and ankles flexed and the chin in. The back is kept straight and usually inclined forward as necessary. The object is positioned between the knees and as close to the body as possible. A good grip is essential and if not readily available the object should be tilted onto one corner and gripped firmly at a free bottom corner on the opposite side. The grip should be performed with the palm of the hand and the roots of the fingers and thumb and not with the fingers alone as they are much weaker. Finally the lift should be performed with the leg muscles. The load is set down by repeating these steps in reverse. The worker must avoid twisting the back throughout the lift, the carry, and the set-down.

The load should be held close to the body or even over the back but always keeping the spine straight. A heavy load at arms' length, particularly if it is to be lifted above the shoulders, often leads to trouble. Practical demonstrations of lifting techniques are reinforced in industry by safety campaigns and wall posters. There is good evidence from studies in various industries of considerable reductions in the numbers of back injuries by use of this kinetic handling technique. In

FIG. 18. Upright posture with load

133

those factories adopting the best handling methods the back injury rate has fallen by up to 50 per cent illustrating the potential benefits.

Unfortunately this advice has failed to make much impact on the back problem as a whole. This is probably because only a tiny proportion of the working population are properly taught the kinetic method of lifting. The number of qualified instructors is very small. Appreciation of the benefits of this handling method should lead to rapidly expanding training programmes.

There are improvements in the design of containers. The primary purpose of a container is to protect the product within. Today thought is also given to how it will be handled. If it is to be lifted then its size, shape, and total weight are important. Ergonomists are designing improvements in the type and position of handles and grips and even the texture of the surface.

Seating

Chairs should be designed for comfort. However, some of the worst back problems arise in those who have to sit all day, particularly at work. Commonly these are caused by poorly designed chairs and would be prevented by better seating. Much research has been devoted to improving the design of chairs but most has been directed at chairs used in offices rather than for domestic purposes. This is probably because the costs involved in developing and manufacturing well-designed products put them out of the reach of the average domestic purchaser. Also one might cynically think that back problems due to poor seating make workers less efficient so that it is economically viable to spend more on the purchase of better chairs. Nevertheless, the principles established in the design of better office furniture apply equally to chairs purchased for the home and many domestic products now incorporate current ideas about design.

The good chair will feel comfortable if it provides proper

support to the body and a healthy sitting posture. If a chair is the wrong size or shape it will be uncomfortable. For this reason chair designers look to measurements of the human frame in order to determine the dimensions of their chairs. However, they do not make a chair specifically designed for the mythical average man as so few of us are actually of that size. Rather, they choose dimensions that will fit a large proportion, usually 90 per cent, of the population. Sometimes this is by having adjustments available on the chair or on other occasions simply by allowing a certain amount of leeway. A chair that would exactly fit the human body would not be tolerable for more than relatively short periods. We all change our posture regularly and frequently during any sitting period. If there is too much control, only a single position could be adopted and this would rapidly produce fatigue. A definition of a good chair is 'one which permits of as many good postures being adopted as possible without interference with the work'.

When sitting, the weight of the trunk is taken mainly by the ischial tuberosities which are the twin bones within the buttocks which can be felt when sitting on a hard surface. They are specially adapted for this purpose and it is normal that they take most of the weight when sitting rather than the surrounding softer and more sensitive tissues. The skin over the two ischial tuberosities is thicker than that covering the rest of the body, with the exception of the soles of the feet, which also have to carry a lot of weight. If the material of a seat is too soft then the pressure is not borne by these bones but is spread out over the whole of the buttocks compressing the skin, muscle, nerves, and blood vessels and this can cause numbness, tingling, and loss of feeling. This is why a seat that is too soft is uncomfortable. A seat exactly contoured to the shape of the buttocks would also be uncomfortable as the weight of the body would be borne by these soft tissues. The seat should be fairly flat with a small amount of upholstery but be firm so that the pressure is concentrated around these bones. It is for this reason that canvas seats are

135

uncomfortable. Their reputation as 'numb bum' seats is due to the spreading of the load widely over the soft tissues.

To compensate for the firmness of the seat, in office chairs springing is often provided in the centre column. This may have a mechanism such as a gas cylinder which can absorb sudden shocks when sitting down and prevent the jarring which would otherwise occur. Such a mechanism also allows for adjustment of the height of the seat. The material in which the seat is upholstered should be porous to avoid the sweating which develops with impermeable materials.

The height of the seat should allow the user to place the soles of his shoes on the floor in comfort. There should be no pressure on the backs of the thighs with the feet resting squarely on the floor. If the seat is too high blood vessels and nerves become pinched resulting in numbness, tingling, and extreme discomfort. The recommended measurements are that the seat height should be slightly less than the height of the underside of the thigh in the seating position. A seat that is low can also cause problems. The hips and knees will be excessively flexed and the sitter will not be able to maintain the normal hollowing of the lower back. He may be forced to adopt a posture involving bending forwards and this commonly produces many back problems.

The depth of the seat should be about 16–21 cm (6–8 in) less than the distance from the back of the buttocks to behind the knee. If the seat is too long it will press on the back of the calf and produce discomfort. The person will be forced to slide forwards to relieve this pressure and will lose the benefit of the back-rest. Seats for use in crowded places and for very short periods may be very shallow. They should be deep enough so that the twin bones, the ischial tuberosities, can rest upon them. If shorter than this no support will be provided.

Most seats are perfectly horizontal. This is the most useful position although a slight backward slope will allow full use of the back-rest. The width of the chair seems less important. Usually they are made wide enough for the broadest person likely to use them to sit in comfort.

Prevention of back pain

When sitting on a stool, the muscles of the back, particularly in the lumbar region, will contract in order to maintain the upright posture. Indeed they are probably more active in this position than when standing. Such continuous muscle activity is tiring. In the absence of a back rest the weight of the trunk may be taken by leaning forward and resting with the arms on a table or by slumping the trunk into the round back position. The strain is born by the ligaments of the spine and this can produce back pain.

A back rest must be strong enough to support the trunk and yet allow movement of the spinal column and of the arms. It does not have to be rigid. A stiff sprung support can be extremely comfortable. The aim of the back rest is to provide a relaxed position with support of the spine in the lumbar region. With a correctly designed lumbar rest, support higher up is unnecessary. The high backs found in some executive chairs are imposing but do not have an important function. The back rest should provide support in the lumbar region below the level of the shoulder blades. If it is too high when the subject relaxes the lumbar muscles slump and the subject sits with the low back bent forwards – a potent cause of back problems. If the back rest is too low it will come into contact with the sacrum or tail bone and push the occupant of the chair forward on the seat. The lower edge of the lumbar support must therefore clear the sacral region. In typists' chairs, the position of the support is adjustable.

The angle of slope of the back-rest of the chair depends very much on the purpose of the seat. The alert position for a secretary is more upright than the comfort position of her boss. Some chairs will have a tilt mechanism so that the occupant can relax lying backwards in the chair. The mechanism must be sprung so that it does not tilt back too easily.

Arm-rests are far from necessary. If present, however, they should be at the right height. They should be at the level of the elbow when sitting. If lower than this they will not provide adequate support to the elbows and if higher they merely get in the way. The latest designs of office chairs incorporate these ideas and various dimensions can be adjusted for individual comfort. For example, a new range of British chair has been created specifically to minimize back problems, and has power-assisted adjustments of both the angle of the back and of the seat height (Plate 10). There is an Italian range which automatically adjusts to provide optimum support with change in position of the body. When leaning forwards, for example at a desk in order to study documents closely, the seat and back-rest shift forwards automatically, and when relaxing backwards the seat moves forwards but the back-rest tilts backwards (Plate 11).

The same principles apply when choosing an upright chair for use in the home. The height, depth of the seat, amount of cushioning, and provision of a lumbar support are equally relevant. For the back sufferer an upright chair of this type may be the answer as low easy-chairs can be extremely uncomfortable. When buying a chair for home use, pay particular attention to the various points mentioned. Above all, sit in it for a few minutes to see how comfortable it is. Most chairs do not feel too bad when sat in for only a moment or two. One should only be satisfied with the chair if it is still comfortable after more prolonged testing.

Unfortunately the same enthusiasm for the development of office chairs has not gone into the design of armchairs and other easy chairs. Many of these have cushioning that is far too soft and without lumbar support so that the back adopts a rounded position and sooner or later starts to ache. The best chairs are well upholstered with a firm seat. This is tilted backwards so that the user leans against a back-rest in which there is a lumbar support at the appropriate height. A high back can support the head when lying back in the armchair and is of more value than in an upright chair.

In past years, automobiles were notorious for poor seating and people whose jobs depended on a lot of driving, such as salesmen, would develop dreadful back problems as a result. Back pain due to prolonged sitting in a poor posture induced by car seats is a well-recognized hazard of that profession.

Prevention of back pain

Fortunately today we hardly see the bench seats or the hammock shaped seats which had a particular reputation for producing back problems.

Ideally the driver's seat should be designed separately from that of his front seat passenger, but this does not happen in practice. Proper support is required for the driver who is in a working position, whereas a relaxed position is ideal for his accompanying passenger. The driving seat itself should have a firm surface with a slight backward tilt and the back-rest contain a lumbar support at the right height. In some cars the amount of lumbar support is adjustable. The back-rest may also be shaped to provide some lateral support so that the driver is not affected by side-sway. Temporary back-rests are available if the car seat is uncomfortable but although they help to some extent their value is limited.

Much thought has gone into the designs of seating for other special purposes. In aircraft the seating must allow for relatively tight packing of the passengers, room to get in and out, and scope for reclining as well as many of the other points already mentioned. The pilot must not only be in a position of comfort for a long flight but also able easily to grasp a number of controls and read a miriad of instruments.

Tables and desks

The design of seating should not be considered in isolation from the desk, table, or bench at which the occupant is working. A table that is too high or too low will produce stresses on the spine and contribute towards back problems. In the office, the chair and desk should be considered as a single unit so that the proper relationships are maintained (Fig. 19). For clerical work, the desk surface should be at about the level of the elbows when sitting upright, and the arms hanging down. This means that the forearm will be horizontal when writing. A higher desk produces a cramped position and the edge of the desk will press on the forearms. The shoulders will often be raised to bring the elbows and forearms onto

139

FIG. 19. A poor posture (above) and the ideal position for a typist at her desk

the desk and the muscle activity will lead to fatigue. For physical work performed sitting at the bench the worker's elbows should bear the same relation to the work surface as if he were doing the same job standing upright.

The vertical distance between the undersurface of the table and the floor and any foot-rest must allow adequate clearance for the knee and thigh. There should be enough room to allow the occupant to cross his legs with a gap between the chair seat and the undersurface of the table of about 25–30 cm (10 or 12 inches).

Conclusions

It is clear that mechanical factors both cause and aggravate the back problem. Much of this develops during work. An understanding of the physical requirements of various jobs and capabilities of employees, coupled with limitation of excessive physical activity, instruction on appropriate manual handling techniques, and modification of the working environment should limit much of the disability we meet today.

9

Ankylosing spondylitis and related disorders

In this book so far the major emphasis has been on the mechanical problems occurring in the back and how they can be prevented and treated. However, backache may develop for other reasons. Recognition of alternative causes of the problem is always important and that is why the back sufferer should always seek medical advice, particularly when the pain develops for the first time.

Inflammation may occur in the joints of the back. There are a number of possible causes of inflammation but most frequently it is due to the condition known as ankylosing spondylitis. This name is developed from 'ankylosis' which means a stiffening, 'spondyl' which refers to the spine, and 'itis' which is the medical suffix indicating inflammation. In other words it is an inflammatory condition of the spine which may lead to stiffening. An ankylosing spondylitis-like problem can occur in other diseases such as ulcerative colitis, Crohn's disease, psoriasis, Reiter's disease, and some other disorders. Initially these back problems were regarded as separate disorders with similar features but recent advances in the study of how ankylosing spondylitis is inherited indicate a close relationship between them. Each of these disorders can be complicated by features of the others, including not only inflammation of the spine but also other problems. Today these conditions are grouped together as the 'seronegative spondarthritides' which means that the serum in the blood when tested is negative for the rheumatoid factor found in rheumatoid arthritis, and that they involve inflammation of the joints of the spine. This group of disorders is quite separate from rheumatoid arthritis although years ago ankylosing spondylitis was regarded by some specialists as rheumatoid arthritis of the spine. This view is no longer held although true

142

rheumatoid arthritis can on occasions affect the back as well as the joints in the limbs.

Ankylosing spondylitis

In its severe form this condition is easily recognized. There is complete loss of the movements in the joints of the back so that the spine becomes completely rigid. The worst cases are as stiff as a poker so the condition is sometimes known as 'poker back'. However, unlike a poker the posture is not upright. The ankylosing spondylitic often ends up in a characteristic but unfortunate position: intensely round-shouldered with a stoop or kyphosis of the upper part of the back. The patient will stretch his neck backwards in an effort to keep looking forwards and avoid looking at the ground. With proper and early treatment it is usually possible to avoid this long-term picture. That is why the disease should be diagnosed as early as possible and the appropriate treatment programme instituted.

Ankylosing spondylitis has been around for a very long time. The changes can be recognized by examination of skeletons so that archaeological evidence is readily obtained. In the excavations of the Egyptian mummies in the Valley of the Kings there is evidence that the condition existed thousands of years before Christ. In the fifth century Caelius Aurelianus described a patient who was 'afflicted with pain in the nates, moved slowly, and could only bend or stand erect with difficulty'. The Bishop of Cork in the eighteenth century described a man who was completely rigid from his feet to his head. He had a job as a watchman in a sentry box because he could only look in one direction. A nineteenth-century medical book illustrates a case with such severe deformity that the head was pointing not only downwards but also backwards so that the patient could only look behind him between his legs. Fortunately such disasters do not occur today. Even now, however, we see people who have developed rigid spines and poor postures in past years. Once the joints have set, it is difficult to do anything about the problem. With modern treatment most of the long-term stiffness and deformities can be prevented.

The condition most often appears in young men. It usually begins between the ages of 15 and 25 years but can start at both younger and older ages. In any young man with backache the question of ankylosing spondylitis must always be considered first as it is remarkably frequent in this age group. One of the easiest ways to find cases is to enquire about backache in a group of university students or army recruits. The disease is thought to occur about five to ten times as frequently in men than women. Cases do occur in females and they can present some of the most difficult problems. Being female does not exclude a diagnosis of ankylosing spondylitis although it does make it less likely.

There has been slight reticence in quoting the frequency of this condition because modern evidence indicates that mild forms are very much more common than previously appreciated. Many backache sufferers may have a sub-clinical type of ankylosing spondylitis and the diagnosis may be missed for years if not indefinitely. The condition may affect 2 per cent of the whole population which means that in Britain there would be well over a million sufferers. These mild forms occur in equal frequencies in the two sexes in contrast to the male preponderance already cited.

Why is it then that the obvious disease appears so much more common in males? The explanation is far from clear. Possible reasons are (a) that the disease is rather worse in men than women; (b) that males on the whole undertake heavier work than females and so have more problems at work; (c) that men complain more than women; (d) that when the back pain occurs in women it is treated as relatively unimportant and probably due to gynaecological problems in contrast with the 'proper' back pain that males suffer. Whatever the reason for this peculiar conundrum, we now realise that mild ankylosing spondylitis is common in both sexes and a frequent cause of backache although more severe problems are less frequent in women and predominantly occur in males.

Ankylosing spondylitis and related disorders

The inflammation usually starts in the sacro-iliac joints, the pair of joints connecting the sacrum to the pelvis; it gradually spreads up the spine to involve first the lumbar area, then the back of the chest and the neck. Sometimes there is also inflammation of the hips, knees, or feet. The inflammation may affect the lining of the joints but has an important characteristic separating it from rheumatoid arthritis and other types of joint disease. This is the involvement of the attachments of ligaments to bone. Inflammation starts there and heals by forming a tiny knob of new bone. The ligament is still attached to the tip of this knob and further inflammation gives rise to progressive lengthening of the bony protuberance, so eventually the whole ligament may be converted into bone. The end-result is that the joints can no longer move and it is this process that eventually will produce the rigid poker spine. The same type of inflammation can happen to ligaments elsewhere and particularly below and behind the heel where spurs of bone may form.

The initial symptom is of low back stiffness and pain. In the early stages the former predominates with an aching quality which only becomes a proper pain as it gets worse. the symptoms are aggravated by rest and relieved by exercise. It is very characteristic that the patient is wakened in the morning by aching and stiffness in the back. He tosses and turns in bed but eventually is forced to get up and obtain relief by doing a few physical jerks. This may happen in the early hours much to the distress of the patient (and his wife) who are unable to get a good night's sleep.

This pattern of symptoms is described in the Bible. Job was a wealthy merchant whose faith in God was tested by the infliction of all sorts of problems. Amongst these Job describes how 'wearisome nights are appointed to me. When I lie down, I say, when shall I rise and the night be gone? And I am full of tossing to and fro until the dawning of the day . . . and the days of affliction have taken hold upon me. My bones are pierced in me in the night season, and my sinews take no rest.' Clearly he had ankylosing spondylitis.

Back pain: the facts

At this early stage of the disease the back may feel and look normal during the day although some backache may return when the patient is tired. This pattern is in complete contrast with the mechanical types of back pain described earlier in this book in which the pain is made easier by rest and worse following physical exertion. The spondylitic also finds that stiffness and aching return if he sits still for any long period and he finds it better to get up and move about frequently.

In mild ankylosing spondylitis, the movements of the back are preserved, especially by the time the patient is seen by a doctor in the surgery when the early morning stiffness will have worn off. It is only later that more severe stiffness persists throughout the day and examination shows restriction of back movements in all directions including bending forwards, backwards, sideways, and twisting. The normal hollowing in the low back may become lost so the lumbar area appears flat. The spine in the back of the chest is normally curved slightly forwards and this becomes worse so that a stoop develops. At the same time the neck feels stiff and painful and movements are restricted.

As the stiffening spreads through the back the patient experiences increasing difficulty in bending or twisting. If he wishes to look behind he is forced to turn his whole body rather than his head alone. Backing the car can be extremely difficult and in severe cases the driver must rely on mirrors rather than look behind. Eventually the back may become completely solid with no movement possible. One saving grace if this happens is that the pain disappears. Pain occurs only when damaged joints move so that a completely solid spine will be painless. However the disability will persist.

Rarely, patients develop progressive stiffening of the back without much in the way of symptoms. They may develop a completely solid spine without realizing that anything is wrong. This has happened in army officers who are trained to stand bolt upright and get stuck in that particular position without realizing it.

Ankylosing spondylitis and related disorders

The same type of inflammation occurs elsewhere. When the joints connecting the ribs to the spine are involved, their movements are lost with reduction in chest expansion. Fortunately we breathe with our diaphragms as well as the rib cage, or the spondylitic would have considerable problems. Inflammation can also affect the joints in the lower limbs, and most often the hips. Progressive reduction in hip movement alone produces problems but when the spine is stiff as well the combination can rapidly lead to total disability. Providing the lower limbs are unaffected, a stiff back does not interfere with one's ability to walk. Even with stiff hips it is possible to walk about by swinging the trunk. When both hips and back are stiff, however, getting out of a chair and walking about may be impossible. Fortunately this complication is rare. Inflammation may also occur behind the heel at the attachment of the Achilles tendon or under the heel producing 'plantar fasciitis'. There is pain and swelling interfering with walking and making it difficult to find comfortable shoes.

The diagnosis of ankylosing spondylitis is confirmed by an X-ray. The initial changes are found in the two sacro-iliac joints. However in early disease the changes are very subtle and the joints may appear quite normal so that the X-ray cannot be used to exclude the diagnosis. Later, features of ankylosing spondylitis are found in the rest of the spine and indicate the severity of the condition.

Inflammation can develop in other tissues of the body and sometimes precedes the onset of back pain. In the eye the iris, which surrounds the pupil, may become acutely inflamed, so that the eye feels painful and vision becomes blurred. This develops in about a third of patients with ankylosing spondylitis. Those who develop one attack are likely to suffer a recurrence and repeated bouts if not properly treated can permanently damage the iris and lens and interfere with eyesight. Inflammation may also occur in the intestines. These types of chronic inflammation of the bowel are known as ulcerative colitis and Crohn's disease. Careful study of the bowel troubles in spondylitic patients does show that a

147

significant proportion have these problems. Either the back or the bowel troubles may start first so it is not possible to say that one complicates the other but rather that they are associated. Very rarely inflammation may also affect the heart. It may damage the aortic valve the function of which is to ensure that blood leaves the heart in the right direction to pass round the body. The damaged valve may leak, so interfering with the work of the heart. If necessary this valve can be replaced at operation by a heart surgeon. The inflammation can also damage the centre within the heart controlling the rhythm of the heart beat. Abnormal rhythms may also impair heart function.

Treatment

With proper treatment, it should be possible to prevent most of the long-term problems of ankylosing spondylitis. However, the responsibility for this is largely that of the patient himself. The fundamentals of the treatment programme are constant attention to posture to prevent deformities arising and regular physiotherapy and exercise to stop the joints becoming stiff and losing their ranges of movement. The physiotherapy treatment must be done every day and if possible twice a day for at least a quarter of an hour each time. Although this does not sound much it is remarkable how few patients adhere to it. Hours are spent in the pub or watching the television yet excuses are found for never having time for these exercises. Undoubtedly repetitive exercises may seem boring but this is a small price to pay in the fight against deformity and disability. It is not possible to emphasize enough the importance attached to these two aspects – attention to posture and physiotherapy.

Attention to posture means constantly stopping oneself from slouching forward but sitting and standing upright in order to correct this tendency. The tall elegant African girls who balance water jugs on their heads and at the other extreme the girls in finishing schools who are taught deportment

PLATE 8. *(Above)*
Modern acupuncture
for back pain.

PLATE 9.
Transcutaneous
nerve stimulation.

PLATE 10. A modern range of office chairs designed for back comfort (by courtesy of Hille International Ltd).

PLATE 11. The automatic Vertebro chair (by courtesy of Anonima Castelli S.P.A.).

PLATE 12. A very severe example of osteoporosis.

FIG. 20. The upright posture and the slouch of the
ankylosing spondylitic

by walking with books on their heads both stand in the right way. This is the posture that must be preserved. The slouch becomes fixed only too readily.

The exercise regime will usually be taught by the physiotherapist in the first instance. However it is not necessary to be treated by a physiotherapist every day but simply to follow the instructions once they are understood. The exercise programme is aimed at maintaining all the movements of the back and neck including bending forwards, backwards, and sideways, and twisting to both sides. Breathing exercises are included to prevent the restriction of the rib cage. There are exercises for the hips and shoulders and other joints. When performed conscientiously, it is usually possible to prevent most if not all the stiffness that otherwise develops.

Swimming is an excellent exercise and should be encouraged. The breast stroke is particularly good for the shoulders and hips, the crawl for the spine and chest, and the back stroke for all muscle groups. However, ankylosing spondylitics should not perform high diving because of the risks of damaging the neck. Other non-competitive sports should be encouraged but care should be taken in those contact sports in which injury may result. It is easy to damage the inflamed back and in advanced disease the spine, although rigid, is weak and fractures occur readily.

When sitting in a chair there should be a proper support in the lumbar region. The bed should be firm and not sag as described in Chapter 5.

Drugs are very effective in relieving the symptoms, particularly in early disease. However, if used alone they will let the patient slouch and develop spine stiffness and deformities in comfort but do nothing to prevent the development of disability. The spondylitic must appreciate that the treatment does not come from a bottle of tablets. Instead he should use medicines to allow him to perform the exercises more thoroughly. The tablets used are both pain relievers and also control inflammation. Aspirin, indomethacin, the propionic acid derivatives such as ibuprofen, naproxen, ketoprofen and the other non-steroidal anti-inflammatory drugs mentioned in Chapter 6 are all used. If anything, they are better at relieving symptoms in this condition than in the mechanical types of back pain. This is because the inflammatory element is so predominant here. As the symptoms are at their worst in the early morning, it is usually helpful to time the medicines to be most effective then. This ususally means taking the drug last thing before going to sleep. Sometimes they pass through the body so quickly that they lose their effect by the early morning. This can be dealt with by using slow-release preparations in which the active constituent is released over a long period into the intestine for absorption. Alternatively, certain of these drugs can be given as suppositories inserted last thing at night. Again the medicine is absorbed only very slowly over a prolonged period.

In former years, deep X-ray irradiation was used as a form of treatment. It was effective in relieving the immediate problems but in the long run made no difference to the patient's progress. Those who received this treatment carry a slightly increased risk of certain complications so that today radiotherapy is reserved for the most difficult cases. However, it is helpful in dealing with persistent areas of inflammation outside the spine, such as the heel.

Surgery has only a very small part to play. When there is a severe deformity of the spine, correction by taking out a small wedge of bone is possible and can be remarkably successful. However, it is quite a formidable procedure and not undertaken lightly. Replacement of severely damaged hip joints is now almost a routine operation in many orthopaedic departments. This operation, developed by Sir John Charnley in Wrightington, has revolutionized the treatment of hip disease in general and can be very effective for the spondylitic with hip problems.

Back pain: the facts

Ulcerative colitis and Crohn's disease and the spine

In both of these conditions there is persistent inflammation of the intestines and both may be complicated by back problems and arthritis in the limb joints. To explain the difference between ulcerative colitis and Crohn's disease, it is necessary to understand the functions of the different parts of the bowels. Food, when swallowed, passes into the stomach where it is mixed up with various digestive juices and then passed into the small intestine where the nutritional parts are absorbed. The remaining debris passes into the large intestine from where it is excreted via the anus or back passage. In ulcerative colitis there is inflammation of the large intestine only, whereas Crohn's disease can affect either or both the small and large intestines. The details of the types of inflammation differ between the two conditions. However both produce recurrent and unpleasant diarrhoea, weight loss, and general ill health.

The inflammation of the back involves the sacro-iliac joints and the rest of the spine in the same way as ankylosing spondylitis. If a patient with ulcerative colitis or Crohn's disease gets backache then this diagnosis should be suspected. Although the bowel and back inflammation can occur together their relationship is not very clear. The bowel disease may be very mild and the back severe and vice versa. Either may occur first. On occasions the link may not be direct in the same patient, but in a close relative. One has bowel problems and the other the ankylosing spondylitis. So it seems that the association depends principally on inherited genetic factors making the two run together rather than one being a direct complication of the other. A particular inherited tissue type predisposes towards ankylosing spondylitis. If a patient with bowel inflammation has this tissue type then his chances of developing spondylitis will be greatly increased. Recent studies have shown that certain types of bacterial infection of the intestine, quite different from ulcerative colitis and Crohn's disease, can also be associated with spondylitis in genetically susceptible individuals.

Ankylosing spondylitis and related disorders

If the back pain is due to spondylitis, then the treatment is the same as in the straightforward condition. However, patients with chronic diarrhoea may have difficulty with the suppositories mentioned and prefer taking these drugs by mouth.

Psoriasis and the back

Psoriasis is a very common persistent skin condition which produces a characteristic rash. There are patches of red thickened skin which if scratched gently will produce a myriad of tiny silver flakes. The rash usually develops over the backs of the elbows, the knees, and the scalp. However it may occur anywhere on the trunk and in severe cases may involve the whole body. Even the skin in apparently unaffected areas shows changes on microscopic examination and the cells are multiplying at a far greater rate than normal. The effects of psoriasis often last for many years although modern treatment usually keeps it under excellent control.

Like inflammatory bowel disease, psoriasis may be associated with disease of the spine and also arthritis in the limb joints. The back problem affects the sacro-iliac joints and the spine in just the same way as ankylosing spondylitis. There is stiffness, low back pain, and progressive development of a stoop and loss of movement and in severe cases permanent deformities of the spondylitic type. Again, inherited factors play an important role in determining whether spondylitis develops. Those psoriatics who are born with the particular tissue type are at special risk of this complication. The treatment of spondylitis in a psoriatic patient is exactly the same as that of ankylosing spondylitis by itself as described earlier.

Reiter's disease

This disorder is named after Hans Reiter, who described in 1916 the illness in a Prussian cavalry officer serving in the Balkans. He developed arthritis following a discharge from the penis and inflammation of the eyes. As with many illnesses

153

named after an individual, the honour of the name seems arbitrary and unfair because the true credit belongs to Sir Benjamin Brodie, an Englishman, who described the disease in 1818. The correct name should be Brodie's disease.

In this country, Reiter's disease most often occurs as a form of venereal disease, particularly in those who are sexually promiscuous. However, this is not always true and in some it develops following infective diarrhoea; outbreaks have been described in closed communities on ships following a form of food poisoning. In certain cases there is no obvious precipitating cause.

The disease usually starts in young adult males but younger and older men and the female sex are not exempt. The first symptom is burning pain on passing urine and the desire to do this much more frequently than normal, although the actual volume passed may be very small. The sensation may waken the patient several times during the night in order to provide relief. A discharge from the penis is common and often seen on first getting out of bed. The patient should be referred to a special venereal disease clinic as various types of infection can cause these symptoms and it is important that the right treatment is instituted before any damage is done. For example, antibiotics are required for gonorrhoea, and syphilis. In Reiter's disease a swab taken from the penis for culture is often sterile. This is called non-specific urethritis or NSU. A week or two later inflammation develops in the eyes and then in the joints. The arthritis usually starts in the feet and knees but sometimes elsewhere. There may be ulcers on the penis or inside the mouth, a rash on the soles of the feet and the rest of the body and other problems.

The back usually is not affected in the first bout of Reiter's disease. However, these patients often develop recurrent attacks without any obvious precipitating cause, and in subsequent bouts the disease may involve the sacro-iliac joints and the spine in the same way as in ankylosing spondylitis. The symptoms of back pain, the limitation of movement, and the deformity are all very similar. Those patients who develop back problems commonly have the same inheritance factor as the spondylitic, illustrating the links between these conditions. Moreover, the rash is very similar to that of psoriasis described earlier.

The treatment of the back problem in Reiter's disease is the same as that of ankylosing spondylitis but in addition in early disease antibiotics are usually prescribed for the NSU. The other features mentioned may also require treatment.

The interrelationships of these conditions

Although these various diseases are described separately it is clear that there is a common strand running through them in that they are all associated with similar types of spine involvement. They have an important link with an inherited tissue type. We are all familiar with the typing of red blood cells into A, B, AB, and O groups which is necessary for patients about to have a blood transfusion. Using blood of the wrong group can provoke severe reactions. The white cells in the blood can be typed in a similar fashion and these are known as the human lymphocyte antigens or HLA antigens. Knowledge of these is important for matching donors and recipients when transplants of organs such as the kidney or heart are considered. Accurate matching is essential to avoid rejection.

One of these tissue types is known as HLA B27. In 1973 workers in the Westminster Hospital in London and the University of California in Los Angeles in the United States simultaneously discovered that this tissue type is present in only about 8 per cent of the general population but 95 per cent of those patients with ankylosing spondylitis. This is the inherited factor predisposing towards ankylosing spondylitis. If you are born with tissue type HLA B27 the risk of developing ankylosing spondylitis is increased about 600 times. In Reiter's syndrome there is the same very close association with HLA B27. The patients with psoriasis, ulcerative colitis, and Crohn's disease who develop ankylosing spondylitis also have a very considerable increase in the incidence of this tissue type.

The reason why inflammation of the spine should be associated with a particular blood cell type is unknown and open to much speculation. One suggestion is that the inheritance gene for spondylitis is located next to that for HLA B27 so that the two tend to be inherited by the same individual. The receptors that determine white blood cell type are located on the surface of the cells. The HLA B27 receptor is structurally very similar to that of certain bacteria. This might mean that the body does not recognize these bacteria as invasive organisms and therefore fails to eliminate them, so they can settle in the spine and produce inflammation. It is still early days to know the answer to this problem.

The seronegative spondarthritides provide an interesting contrast to the mechanical problems described earlier in this book. Although seemingly separate these various conditions possess complex and fascinating interrelations with each other.

10

Some other back problems

The preceding chapters have covered the more common back problems. However, a number of other disorders may be responsible for back pain. Some can lead to severe damage of the spine if left untreated. They are described in this chapter in order to emphasize the need for skilled medical advice in elucidating back problems. This is particularly important when the pain develops for the first time and if it does not repeat a pattern which has occurred before.

Infections in the back

Infections are due to germs which are usually bacteria or viruses. Bacteria are minute single-celled living organisms that can invade and multiply in the tissues. An infection in the skin produces inflammation and if pus is formed it becomes an abscess. Occasionally bacterial infections occur in the bones of the spine causing osteomyelitis, and if pus develops a spinal abscess forms. The infection has usually spread to the back from elsewhere in the body, such as a boil in the skin. Back pain gradually develops and becomes extremely severe. The patient feels ill and develops a high temperature and often shivering attacks. This is quite different from the types of backache previously mentioned. The treatment involves identifying the particular bacteria and treating it with the right antibiotic. Occasionally a surgeon may drain the pus from a spinal abscess.

Tuberculosis is another example of infection. It usually occurs in the lungs. Bone tuberculosis is usually due to drinking milk from infected cattle. In the back the disease is known as 'Pott's disease' after Sir Percival Pott (1713–88). In the past tuberculosis of the spine was a dreaded complication

157

because the infection could severely damage the bones and nerves. With pasteurization of milk and testing of cattle, tuberculosis of the spine is now relatively rare although surprisingly there has been some increase in frequency in the last few years. Modern treatment is remarkably effective in dealing with this condition but it should be started as soon as possible to limit spinal damage.

Another type of bacterial infection affecting the back is brucellosis or undulant fever. This infection is transmitted in milk from cows and currently there is an extensive campaign to eliminate brucellosis from dairy herds. Unfortunately this is not as easy as the elimination of tuberculosis and there is a small risk for those who drink unpasteurized milk from cows that are not brucellosis free. Veterinary surgeons are at particular risk of developing this infection because of their close contact with cattle.

Viruses do not affect the bones but one virus, that of shingles or herpes zoster, can affect the lumbar nerve roots. Pain develops both in the back and in the lower limb in the area supplied by the nerve and for several days the problem can resemble mechanical types of back pain and sciatica. However, after a week or so the virus produces a rash in the area supplied by the particular nerve root and this gives the correct diagnosis.

Rheumatoid arthritis and the back

Rheumatoid arthritis is a persistent inflammation of joints, principally in the limbs, which may eventually produce permanent damage and deformities. The diagnosis is usually obvious in more severe cases.

Occasionally the disease affects the spine and occurs in both the neck and the lumbar areas. When back pain occurs in rheumatoid patients it is often difficult to know whether it arises because of the mechanical problems that are described earlier or to rheumatoid involvement of the joints of the back. Until quite recently it was thought that the disease did not affect the lumbar area but this was mainly because of the difficulties in identifying rheumatoid changes on X-rays of the low back. With modern techniques we now believe that this is much more common than previously thought. The treatment is the same as for rheumatoid arthritis elsewhere.

Diseases of the bone

Bone is not a uniform strengthening material like a steel strut but has a complicated structure. It consists of a dense outer sheath enclosing a meshwork of tough fibres. These fibres are made of tissue somewhat similar to that of the ligaments but strengthened by crystals of a mineral called calcium hydroxy-apatite which are packed into the fibres like tiny bricks. The calcium in bones comes from our food and is absorbed from the intestine, provided there is sufficient vitamin D. Both calcium and vitamin D come from dairy products such as milk, butter, and eggs, but vitamin D is also formed directly in the skin by exposure to sunlight.

If there is an inadequate fibrous framework, only a limited amount of calcium can be laid down. The bone is very weak and this is known as osteoporosis. It is common in older people and particularly women. It may develop as a result of certain diseases and taking cortisone and similar drugs for a long time. In another disorder, osteomalacia, the fibrous framework may be formed normally but insufficient calcium is laid down so that the soft tissue is not changed into proper bone. The principal reason is a lack of vitamin D in the diet, particularly in those who live in overcrowded slum areas where there is little sunlight. In Britain, osteomalacia most often affects Asian immigrants but also is seen in the elderly who rarely go out of doors and live on an inadequate diet. Lack of calcium can be due to a chemical called phytic acid which combines with calcium in the food making it unavail-able for the bones. Phytic acid is present in bread but for-tunately is destroyed during fermentation. However, it persists in unleavened bread such as chapatis and may be

FIG. 21. The structure of the bone of the spine and
the changes in osteoporosis and osteomalacia

160

partly responsible for the osteomalacia in Asian immigrants. A recent trial of chapati-free diets led to a significant improvement in the calcium in their bones.

Lack of calcium and vitamin D can be due to disorders of the intestines. In certain diseases failure to absorb food constituents normally can produce osteomalacia and other disorders. In some this is due to a sensitivity of the bowel to gluten, a protein present in wheat. Simply eliminating gluten from the diet may be enough to control the problem.

In both osteoporosis and osteomalacia there is progressive weakness of the bones. In the spine a stoop may gradually develop because the bone in the vertebrae gives way, causing frequent small fractures. Each time a fracture occurs there may be intense pain which gradually gets better over a few days as the fracture heals. These are known as 'crush' fractures and the sufferer may gradually become round-shouldered and lose height as a result. This is the reason why old people often grow shorter (Plate 12).

Careful testing is needed to distinguish osteoporosis and osteomalacia and determine whether there is any underlying cause. Appropriate treatment is then instituted. Calcium and vitamin D will probably be required but the dose given must be carefully controlled as too much can also do harm. A new preparation known as microcrystalline calcium hydroxy-apatite (Ossopan) is currently under test and looks promising for these conditions.

An acute attack of pain in the back is probably due to a small fracture. During the painful period the sufferer rests in bed, giving the fracture a chance to heal. He is able to get up after a few days; the rest should not be too long as immobility itself weakens the bones.

Paget's disease

In this condition there is excessive formation and turnover of bone. It was described by Sir James Paget who lived from 1814 to 1899. The disease occurs in all countries but with enormous variations in frequency and there is now a strong suggestion that it is caused by a virus infection in the bone. One common site for Paget's disease is the bones of the back. The bones become enlarged and deformed and painful. Until recently little could be done other than providing simple pain-relieving tablets but recent research has produced drugs that are extremely effective not only in controlling the pain, but also in correcting the bony changes.

Tumours in the spine

Fortunately these tumours are rare. A spinal tumour may be a primary growth or secondary to disease in other organs. The tumour may be benign which means that it does not spread, grows very slowly, and if removed will not recur. However, it can also be due to a malignant cancer or occasionally to leukaemia and Hogkin's disease. A tumour causes pain in the back. If the nerve roots are damaged there may be weakness and loss of sensation in the legs or the lower part of the body. Careful examination and tests are needed to make the right diagnosis. Treatment with medicines, surgery, or X-rays may be required and can be remarkably effective.

Back pain in pregnancy

The mechanical weight of the baby in the womb alters the centre of gravity of the mother's body. The ligaments of the pelvis are looser than usual so that the normal lumbar hollow-ing increases, causing strains on the ligaments of the spine. Low back pain is common. The joints of the pelvis separate just before birth to allow the baby to pass through safely during delivery. As a result the sacro-iliac joints may become tender and painful.

The best advice to the mother is to have adequate periods of rest in a properly supported bed, to avoid putting on too much weight, and to wear a pelvic support. The vast majority of back pains of this type recover completely following

Some other back problems

delivery but on occasions the loose sacro-iliac joints do not close completely and persistent pain results. A firm pelvic binder is usually all that is required.

Referred pain

When pain is felt in the back it has not necessarily originated there. This concept has been discussed previously: pain can be felt in the leg due to a burst disc in the spine. Equally, disorders within the abdomen and pelvis can be felt as pain in the back. In particular peptic ulcers, inflammation of the pancreas, and various types of gynaecological disorders can produce back pain. Generally there are features of the problem to indicate their source. Examination of the abdomen or pelvis will reveal tender areas and pressure will produce back pain. With gynaecological problems the pain is often related to the time of the periods. Moreover the back itself is not tender and movements do not exacerbate the symptoms.

11

Social, psychological, and psychiatric aspects of back pain

Of all the difficulties in dealing with back pain, these aspects present perhaps the greatest and most challenging problems. The interaction of organic disease and behaviour is difficult to understand even for straightforward medical problems where the actual physical cause is known. In patients suffering from back pain, we often do not know whether it all arises because of disorders in the back, whether it is entirely a psychological problem, or whether the two interact in some complex fashion. Nevertheless, the patient's pain is every bit as painful whether it is due to organic disease in the spine or develops entirely in the mind. There is a great tendency to think that psychogenic pain is imaginary and not real, in contrast to pain due to a physical illness that requires treatment. All pain is felt in the mind, however it is caused. If anything, the pain associated with psychological and psychiatric disturbances can be worse than that of organic disease alone. A sympathetic and proper understanding of the nature of the problem can lead to a constructive plan of treatment.

We all react in different ways to adversity. Some will tolerate unpleasant events with little emotional reaction while other suffer considerably. These differing psychological reactions occur in the back pain patient and an essential part of the clinical assessment is to determine the role of the mind in the interpretation of individual symptoms.

Malingering and compensation neurosis

Perhaps the simplest problem is that of the malingerer – the person who deliberately pretends he has pain in order to avoid something unpleasant or else to obtain some benefit. Obvious

164

examples are children who complain of a tummy-ache or back pain in order to avoid going to school, or a worker who wants a day off in order to watch a football match. No amount of treatment to the back could make any difference here. Although this type of malingering does occur, it is probably far less common than newspapers would have us believe. It is easy to exaggerate the importance of this problem. It may account for the odd day off but deliberate pretence of back pain by and large does not cause persistent disability.

Doubt is often thrown on the veracity of a patient's statement about back pain if the symptoms follow an accident and there is to be legal action to obtain compensation. One often hears both doctors and lawyers say that such patients will fail to get better until they have received their compensation, and that once the settlement is achieved the pain will disappear without treatment. This is called a compensation neurosis. The symptoms are either fabricated or develop subconsciously because of the financial benefit to be obtained. A diagnosis of compensation neurosis is often invoked in such patients when there are no definite clinical findings to explain the symptoms. There is suspicion on the part of the doctor that he finds difficult to conceal. The patient attempts to convince the sceptical physician and may exaggerate his symptoms, so making the diagnosis and treatment more difficult. The end-result is mutual distrust and persistence of the problem.

Although these views about compensation neurosis are held so widely, there is virtually no evidence in their support. There is no information of the effects of settling legal claims of back pain patients but a study of a similar problem of persistent headache after head injury failed to find any effect of compensation on the outcome. It is true that following a back injury the persistent pain can be due to a combination of the actual damage and psychological factors, but to simplify the problem as just being 'after the money' is a gross misrepresentation of the position. It can impugn the motives of patients when no justification exists. There may be damage

165

in the spine not demonstrable by routine tests which could explain all the problems. Moreover the psychological reactions of normal people following an accident can be just as much an injury as an actual fracture or laceration. If the shock produces an anxiety state or depression this should be considered in the same way as physical damage. Legal minds try to disentangle the actual effects of the accident from the patient's previous condition. If someone already has backache and becomes a bit worse after an accident, his compensation will be very different from that awarded to someone with a previously normal back. A weakness in the back, putting it at greater risk, would also be taken into account. Likewise, his previous mental state may well influence the psychological reactions to the accident and may play a crucial part in deciding the outcome. A person who is prone to psychological problems, has an accident, and develops back pain thought to be of psychological origin is likely to receive less compensation than a person whose disability can be blamed on the accident alone.

The effects of accidents, legal claims, and compensation on back pain are worthy of further research.

Psychological aspects of back pain

Some people suffer from pain in the absence of or with minimal disease to account for it. A simplistic view used to be that people born with a particular personality or meeting particular types of problem might develop certain patterns of symptoms. Although there is some truth in this, modern psychological studies indicate a very complex interplay between medical, psychological, and social factors in the development of the patient's response to disease.

Psychological factors are a combination of the subject's inherent personality and experiences during development, particularly childhood. Perhaps the most obvious example of personality influences are those people who have the condition known as alexithymia which means 'without words for feelings'. These people are unable to experience emotional states, particularly if adverse, such as anxiety or anger. Instead, these emotions may be translated into and felt as physical symptoms such as back pain. Alexithymia may be due to a physical abnormality in the brain such as lack of the nerve connections required for experiencing physical emotions, or psychological problems caused for example by abnormal relationships during early development.

Pain is an experience felt in the mind. It is not simply there, but is learned during childhood as a response to various situations. The very small child does not cry because he is slapped but because of the anger expressed by his parents. Only subsequently does he learn to associate the slap with something unpleasant – pain. There are two types of learning or conditioning process that are relevant and analogies drawn from animal studies help us to understand human pain. When a dog sees food it forms profuse saliva in the mouth. If a bell is rung each time the food is offered, the dog will rapidly associate the bell with food and will even salivate when the bell rings alone without food being offered. This involuntary response is known as 'respondent conditioning'. On the other hand 'operant conditioning' occurs when an animal learns to press a bar because this is followed by the presentation of food. This is a voluntary process that has been learned.

Current concepts suggest that the outward expression of pain, such as wincing or crying is an example of operant conditioning. A child does something wrong, feels guilty, and experiences pain as a mechanism to expiate the guilt. It cries and is comforted by its mother. The comforting is a response that the child likes. It learns that crying means additional attention and care from its mother.

The theory is that pain and its outward expression such as complaining, groaning, wincing, etc., are maintained by compensations to the sufferer. This is not a deliberate decision but a subconscious reaction of the mind outside the individual's control. Compensation does not mean only monetary benefit but also other rewards such as sympathy and concern

167

shown by relatives and friends, and being relieved of problems and responsibilities. In other words, there is a 'pay-off' which reinforces behaviour such as complaining about back pain and so encourages it to be repeated. The patient's spouse, family, friends, nurses, and doctors directly reinforce the pain by displaying sympathy, concern, and attention whenever pain is experienced. The patient is given medicines and encouraged to rest while others assume his problems and responsibilities. Indirect reinforcement of pain arises by the patient avoiding those situations that may be thought likely to exacerbate the symptoms. Inactivity, inability to work and social isolation mean that he is unable to earn a living; this progressively results in self-perpetuating invalidism. The patient's spouse or relations may also reinforce dependency and invalidism. They encourage the patient to feel pain, perhaps because of an excessive need to care for an invalid, or even to alleviate their own psychological problems.

As pain behaviour has been maintained and encouraged by these reinforcers, treatment is aimed at reversing the pain–reward situation and altering the patient's behaviour. In some pain clinics, patients whose pain is believed to be caused in this way may be treated by a complex behaviour modification programme using operant conditioning. Normally behaviour associated with pain such as complaining, wincing, groaning, crying, etc., would be treated with concerned attention, sympathy, and drugs which in practice only reinforce the symptoms in these people. In this programme the medical and nursing staff, with the prior full knowledge and consent of the patient and his relatives, ignore displays and if they develop either simply do not comment or discuss some other topic. The relatives and friends must also learn to ignore the illness behaviour and pain displays. Many of these patients are very inactive and behave as semi-invalids. A programme of gradual physical rehabilitation is introduced with specified physical activities each day, gradually increasing over several weeks. Successful performance of the required activities is encouraged and positively reinforced so that hopefully the patient gets back to something like a normal life.

The cynics suggest that this is how most physiotherapy treatment for the back works anyway. The optimism of most physiotherapists combined with encouragement to tackle progressively more difficult tasks and to return to normal physical activity may well be of far more value than the actual treatment itself.

Once it is decided that conventional medicine has nothing to offer, the patient and his relatives must avoid excessive consultations, investigations, prescriptions, and indulgent medical care. Finally, following successful treatment, positive reinforcement of well behaviour must continue to prevent the patient slipping back to his previous state. This may require supervision of retraining and return to work, and special counselling about individual problems.

Operant conditioning is particularly popular in the United States. It is not practised in exactly the same way in all clinics but the principles have been incorporated into various types of treatment programmes. The results are spectacularly successful in some cases but in others can be disappointing.

Personality and back pain

We all think we know what is meant by 'personality'. We recognize people as being of a particular type and think of them as cheerful, extrovert, difficult, and so on. However, these descriptions depend very much on whoever makes them and often there are completely contrasting views on the personality of an individual. The Prime Minister is honest, concerned, and sympathetic; or hard and an inveterate liar, according to one's politics. In an effort to provide more meaningful descriptions of personality, psychologists have developed a number of standard tests as objective measures of personality. These tests involve detailed questionnaires and often appear in very simplified or humorous forms in the newspapers as games or quizzes. These personality inventories have been used to study back pain patients to see if the

chronic pain sufferer has a particular personality trait. Interpretation of the results of these questionnaires is not easy,
especially as comparison between different ones show that
they are not very reliable. However, interesting contrasts in
the personalities of back sufferers arise between those whose
symptoms are caused by a clear-cut and definite disorder
such as a burst disc and those in whom physical examination
and investigation have not found any abnormality. The latter
group show increased scores for hypochondriasis, which is
the imagining of excessive illness, depression, and hysteria. A
form of mental dissociation takes place as there are abnormal
symptoms in the absence of any physical cause. Such patients
are miserable, worried, and tense. They are convinced they
suffer from a deep-seated illness despite evidence to the con-
trary. Their complaints may be the result of inner psychological conflicts and may be reinforced by a 'reward' as previously
described. However, they will deny that their life problems
and personalities affect the back pain in any way.

Can prolonged back pain cause these personality changes?
After all it would not be too difficult to believe that persistent
chronic disabling symptoms that fail to get better after repeated consultations, investigations, medical treatment, and
even operations would leave one miserable and depressed
about the future. Psychologists and psychiatrists have ad-
dressed themselves to this chicken and egg problem of
whether the pain causes personality changes or the abnormal
personality causes the experience of pain. There is no easy
answer but only clues from some recent studies. The psychological indices of patients severely and permanently paralysed
because of poliomyelitis or other similar problems did not
differ from those of normal people. In rheumatoid arthritis,
psychological testing was normal in those with clear-cut
disease but abnormal in those with symptoms but in whom
the diagnosis was less certain. Those back sufferers who have
an abnormal personality are less likely to respond well to
medical or surgical treatment than those with normal personalities. These observations point to the personality having a

Social, psychological, and psychiatric aspects of back pain

fundamental role in the development and perpetuation of chronic illness. However, the question of which comes first may not be useful as the organic disease, the personality, and the pain interact with and build upon one another in complex and ill-understood fashions. What matters is understanding why the problem persists and what to do about it rather than how it started. There is scope for considerable further research.

Anxiety states and back pain

We all know what being anxious means — we feel tense and sweaty and the pulse rate increases. Normally anxiety is due to mental stress experienced for example before taking an examination or making a speech. However, an anxiety state can develop as a psychological problem and produce back pain. In psychiatric terms, an abnormal anxiety state expresses itself in three main forms: as a sense of fear and tension without any obvious cause — this is known as free-floating anxiety; as unwarranted fear of a particular object or situation such as fear of enclosed spaces (claustrophobia); and as a physical symptom such as back pain.

Patients with an anxiety state develop abnormal contractions of the muscles of the trunk which are easily shown by electrical testing. These tense muscles are associated with aches and pains, particularly in the back as well as elsewhere. The muscle contractions are worse whenever anxiety increases and particularly in difficult and unpleasant situations. The patient feels the symptoms in these tense muscles so that the back pain is the result of the chronic anxiety state. Understanding the psychological basis of the problem indicates the treatment. The first step is to identify the physical, social, and psychological stresses that may be responsible for the anxiety state. If these can be eliminated or modified then the problem may resolve. For some patients a tranquillizer may be appropriate particularly if taken for only a short period to cover a period of particular stress. There are medicines that

171

will relax muscles and limit some of the excessive muscle tension occurring in anxiety states. Often they are combined with pain-relieving medicines in a single tablet.

Psychologists have developed various specialized methods for treating patients with anxiety states. In biofeedback, the patient is given a degree of control over the symptoms by learning consciously to control an electrical signal which informs him about the amount of muscle tension. Hypnosis is an ill-understood mental state of heightened suggestibility and sometimes provides better relief from tension than more straightforward treatment. Some patients receive training in relaxation techniques – that is, the achievement of a profound state of both mental and physical relaxation. These treatment methods may be combined with progressive desensitization to factors identified as responsible for the anxiety state. For example, fear of open spaces (agrophobia) can be eliminated by a treatment programme introducing the patient gradually to more and more open environments, combined with relaxation procedures. The technique of operant conditioning has already been described.

Back pain and depression

We all feel depressed if a close friend or relative dies, we fail an examination or some other disaster strikes. However, in psychiatric terms, depression refers to an excessively sad mood that may develop without any obvious cause or that is out of proportion to a relatively trivial or passing problem. Sometimes it may appear as 'masked' depression in which the depression is disguised as bodily symptoms and quite commonly as back pain and sciatica. On casual enquiry, the depression is not obvious and the patient may not be aware of it. However, there may be other features that make the diagnosis clear. In a study of back pain patients a poor response to conventional treatment correlated with a high incidence of depression. Belief that depression causes pain rather than simply being a consequence of persistent back problems has led to the use of anti-depressant drug therapy for such patients. The modern medicines are very successful in treating depression and very helpful for back pain of this cause.

Back pain and sexual problems

Because of the direct and symbolic links of the back with the basic movements involved in sexual intercourse it has been suggested that back disorders may be linked with sexual dysfunction. There is much speculation but little definite evidence about this. The most obvious reason for a loss of interest or a decline in sexual performance is that intercourse produces severe back pain. This can simply be the result of mechanical stress on the spine rather than being due to any psychological causes. In a way this is the easiest problem to deal with as sympathetic understanding by the partner combined with simple practical advice may be all that is required. A firm bed, a board under the mattress, a pillow in the small of the back or a reversal of positions can help enormously. Some back sufferers take pain-relieving tablets about half an hour in advance.

Depression and chronic anxiety states can cause loss of libido and failure to achieve an erection. In its turn this gives rise to further conflict and anxiety, which perpetuates the problem. Often such patients will not discuss their difficulties and so the problem becomes magnified, deep-rooted, and intractable. Appropriate treatment by medical or psychological means can help enormously.

Finally, a pre-existing sexual problem may provide a deliberate or subconscious motive for the complaint of back pain. The impotent husband who injures his back may discover that his pain provides an acceptable excuse for avoiding sex in the same way that the proverbial headache exempts the wife from the unwelcome attentions of her partner.

Management of the psychological aspects of back pain

It is clear that there is a complex interplay between the physical responses to problems in the back and the human mind. A full medical assessment requires the doctor to consider the psychological and social aspects of the problem and if necessary to institute appropriate treatment. This may be a combination of physical treatment with drugs to lessen anxiety and control depression. Assessment of the patient's personality, past and present, and of any stressful events can suggest psychological therapy such as behaviour modification techniques and exploration and adjustment of the patient's social relationships with his family, friends, and work. The relationship between back pain and the mind is complex and must always be considered carefully by those caring for back pain sufferers.

Glossary

acupuncture: a system originally developed in China for relieving pain by insertion of needles into the skin.

ankylosing spondylitis: a disorder most common in young men, producing inflammation in the joints of the spine and occasionally elsewhere, together with back pain. It may lead to progressive stiffness and deformity.

annulus fibrosus: the fibrous outer layer of the intervertebral disc.

chiropractic: a system for manipulation of the spine.

epidural injection: an injection into the vertebral canal. Local anaesthetic and cortisone are used in this way to relieve the symptoms of back pain.

HLA B27: the white cell type that predisposes to the development of ankylosing spondylitis.

intervertebral disc: the flat cushion which lies between the bodies of the vertebrae.

kinetic handling techniques: manual methods of lifting and carrying heavy objects which minimize the risk of injury to the back.

kyphosis: an unnatural forward angulation of the spine.

lumbago: an acute attack of pain in the lumbar region.

manipulation: treatment of back pain by manual pressure.

nucleus pulposus: the gelatinous (jelly-like) centre of the intervertebral disc.

osteopathy: a form of manipulation of the back which is used by certain medical and non-medical practitioners.

osteomalacia: weakness of the bones because of calcium deficiency. It may be due to poor diet, lack of sunlight, or failure to absorb nutrients and vitamins properly from the bowel.

osteoporosis: weakness of the bones due to a deficient fibrous framework. It may occur in older people, particularly women, as a result of certain diseases, and after taking certain drugs.

175

Back pain: the facts

prolapsed intervertebral disc: a burst of the disc backwards and usually to one side or the other, producing damage to nerve roots and the symptoms of pain in the back and the lower limb.

sciatica: pain felt in the back of the thigh and in the leg due to damage of the nerve roots by a burst intervertebral disc.

slipped disc: a misnomer for a prolapsed intervertebral disc.

spinal stenosis: narrowing of the vertebral canal so that the nerve roots are at greater risk of damage.

spondylosis: wear and tear damage of the spine.

transcutaneous nerve stimulation: an electrical method of stimulating the back which may reduce the sensation of pain in a similar fashion to acupuncture.

trigger points: localized areas of extreme tenderness in the back.

vertebra: one of the elements making up the spinal column.

List of organizations for back pain patients

Below are listed some of the national and international societies and organizations which are concerned with back pain. These bodies will be pleased to offer advice, information, and assistance. However, they are only able to deal with enquiries in general terms. For individual problems patients should refer to their own family doctor and the specialist and paramedical services at his disposal.

Arthritis and Rheumatism Council
41 Eagle Street, London WC1R 4AR.

Back Pain Association
Grundy House, Somerset Road, Teddington, Middx. TW11 8TD

British Rheumatism and Arthritis Association
6 Grosvenor Crescent, London SW1X 7ER

National Ankylosing Spondylitis Society
c/o: Royal National Hospital for Rheumatic Disease, Bath

European League Against Rheumatism
Oberwilerstrasse 23, Postach 146, CH-4011 Basle, Switzerland

International League Against Rheumatism
B.P. 145, CH-4011 Basle, Switzerland

Arthritis Foundation
3400 Peachtree Road, N.E., Atlanta, Georgia 30326, USA

Australian Arthritis and Rheumatism Foundation
Box 144 GPO, Sydney, New South Wales 2001, Australia.

Index

Index

Index

transcutaneous nerve stimulation 104, 109–10
trigger points 111–12
tumours 162

ulcerative colitis 142, 147, 152–3
ultrasound scan 55

vertebrae 8
    structure of 8

vertebral column 2, 6–14
    structure of 2–3
vertebral slips 48

wear and tear, effects of 41
    X-ray diagnosis of 43–5

X-rays 39, 43–5
    use in pre-employment screening 115